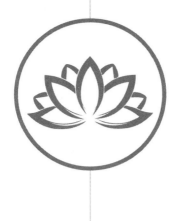

Yoga Therapy

A Personalized Approach
for Your Active Lifestyle

contents

part I   Fundamentals of Yoga Therapy

part II   Foundations of Practice

Yoga Therapy

A Personalized Approach for Your Active Lifestyle

Kristen Butera
Staffan Elgelid

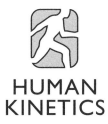

HUMAN KINETICS

Library of Congress Cataloging-in-Publication Data

Names: Butera, Kristen, 1974- author. | Elgelid, Staffan, author.
Title: Yoga therapy : a personalized approach for your active lifestyle /
    Kristen Butera, Staffan Elgelid.
Description: Champaign, IL : Human Kinetics, 2017.
Identifiers: LCCN 2016049236 (print) | LCCN 2016051572 (ebook) (print) |
    LCCN 2016051572 (ebook) | ISBN 9781492529200 (print) | ISBN 9781492531388
    (ebook)
Subjects: LCSH: Hatha yoga--Therapeutic use.
Classification: LCC RM727.Y64 B888 2017 (print) | LCC RM727.Y64 (ebook) | DDC
    613.7/046--dc23
LC record available at https://lccn.loc.gov/2016049236

ISBN: 978-1-4925-2920-0 (print)

This publication is written and published to provide accurate and authoritative information relevant to the subject matter presented. It is published and sold with the understanding that the author and publisher are not engaged in rendering legal, medical, or other professional services by reason of their authorship or publication of this work. If medical or other expert assistance is required, the services of a competent professional person should be sought.

The web addresses cited in this text were current as of November 2016, unless otherwise noted.

Acquisitions Editor: Michelle Maloney; **Developmental Editor:** Tom Heine; **Managing Editors:** Tom Heine and Nicole Moore; **Copyeditor:** Annette Pierce; **Permissions Manager:** Martha Gullo; **Senior Graphic Designer:** Nancy Rasmus; **Cover Designer:** Keith Blomberg; **Photograph (cover):** es/Getty Images/iStockphoto; **Photographs (interior):** Neil Bernstein, unless otherwise noted; **Photo Asset Manager:** Laura Fitch; **Visual Production Assistant:** Joyce Brumfield; **Photo Production Manager:** Jason Allen; **Senior Art Manager:** Kelly Hendren; **Illustrations:** © Human Kinetics; **Printer:** Sheridan Books;

We thank the YogaLife Institute in Wayne, Pennsylvania, for assistance in providing the location for the photo shoot for this book.

Human Kinetics books are available at special discounts for bulk purchase. Special editions or book excerpts can also be created to specification. For details, contact the Special Sales Manager at Human Kinetics.

Printed in the United States of America   10 9 8 7 6 5 4 3 2 1

The paper in this book is certified under a sustainable forestry program.

Human Kinetics

Website: www.HumanKinetics.com

United States: Human Kinetics
P.O. Box 576
Champaign, IL 61825-5076
800-747-4457
e-mail: info@hkusa.com

Canada: Human Kinetics
475 Devonshire Road Unit 100
Windsor, ON N8Y 2L5
800-465-7301 (in Canada only)
e-mail: info@hkcanada.com

Europe: Human Kinetics
107 Bradford Road
Stanningley
Leeds LS28 6AT, United Kingdom
+44 (0) 113 255 5665
e-mail: hk@hkeurope.com

E6772

acknowledgments

From Kristen

Writing a book is no joke. I first witnessed and participated in the process years ago when I edited my husband's books, *The Pure Heart of Yoga* and *Meditation for Your Life*. In general, writing takes a serious willingness to explore yourself and your ideas. Then it takes time, patience, prayer, revisions, and more time. It also takes a village of support and love, which I had in spades. That means that I have a lot of gratitude to express!

My Family and Friends

Writing a book can sometimes be an exercise in being alone. For the grace that they gave me in terms of extra time, I have to thank my family and friends for being loving and supportive forces in my life, giving me the space that I needed to work on the project, patiently missing me, and listening to my challenges as I sorted through the process of writing. I especially want thank my husband, Bob Butera, for his ongoing kindness, patience, and encouragement.

My Colleagues

Thank you to my writing colleague, Staffan Elgelid, for the incredible experiences we had together collaborating on this work over the last 5 years. Our paths intersected at just the right time, and our interactions have changed the way I think about and see the world. I look forward to continued collaborations and explorations in the years to come.

Thank you to my colleague and friend Erin Byron, who worked as a content editor. Her enthusiasm and tireless championing of the work has been an ongoing source of inspiration to me. The guidance and insights she brought to the writing process were invaluable, and the final product was very much improved as a result of all of her contributions.

The Team at Human Kinetics

My thanks to the team at Human Kinetics. Acquisitions editor Michelle Maloney asked for a manuscript proposal at just the right time. Her willingness to discuss and explore our interests ignited the potential themes of the book, and her belief in the value of our work made the book possible. Developmental editor Tom Heine's insightful comments and attention to all of the details shaped the structure of the work. Photographer Neil Bernstein's keen eye brought it all to life in pictures. I know that there are even more people behind the scenes who came together to help bring our vision into reality, and I thank you all.

To My Significant Teachers

When you accumulate the amount of yoga education that I have over the years, you owe a debt of gratitude to all who forged that path of expansion of yoga in the West. There have been many teachers over the years to whom I am grateful, but a few stand out as having helped me become who I am today. Darlene DePasquale helped me create the foundations of my practice and inspired me to become a teacher. Trailblazer Paul Grilley introduced me to the concept of structural variety and changed my approach early on in my teaching journey. Gil Hedley helped me to connect the study of anatomy to a sense of sacred inner knowing. Movement maven Jill Miller profoundly inspired my leadership and movement skills at a crucial time in my personal and professional development. Bill Harvey guided my somatic journey and helped me to integrate my experience of self. My extraordinary husband, Bob Butera, continues to be my greatest teacher. His commitment to our marriage and the work that we do together in the world has given me a true partner on the path of enlightenment.

The YogaLife Institute Community

As the book was being written, we moved our beloved YogaLife Institute studio. So many people helped us clean, pack, move, unpack, and pull the new location together. The contribution of the YogaLife community offered support during a time of tremendous transition for me. The work they do keeps YogaLife a thriving hub of consciousness and transformation, and for that I am eternally grateful.

In particular, senior teachers Libby Piper, Erika Tenenbaum, and Jennifer Hilbert were early readers of the manuscript as well as early adopters and contributors to the developing methodology. Collaborating with them is one of the great joys of my life. The YogaLife studio manager, Erica Saellam, helps keep all of the trains running on time, and her hard work and dedication improve everything that she touches.

Asana models Erin Byron, Al Cochrane, Derek Hopkins, and Libby Piper brought a tremendous amount of positive energy into the photo shoot sessions. Working with them was a joy, and the quality of the photos in the book was expanded by their clear intentions and contributions.

And finally, a huge offering of gratitude goes out to anyone and everyone who has participated in my classes, trainings, seminars, and asana labs over the years. Your dedication and willingness to learn and explore continually inspires, uplifts, and drives me forward. Seeing you discover your potential, and then share it with others, makes me feel like I am on the side of the angels. Many blessings to you all!

From Staffan

I doubt that anyone who has written a book can thank all of the people who have helped in various ways. There simply isn't enough space to thank everyone. The people I will mention are just a fraction of all who have supported me.

First, I want to thank my coauthor, Kristen Butera. It was a pleasure seeing our ideas move from the yoga studio to the page, back to the studio for refinement, and then back to the page in refined form. What a joy to muck around with the concepts until we felt that they were ready to be written down. I am looking forward to continued mucking around with you and bringing these concepts to a bigger audience.

To the people at Human Kinetics, you have all given us amazing support. Thanks, Michelle Maloney, for contacting Kristen and getting the book off the ground. Thanks to Tom Heine for editing and editing and editing. You did a phenomenal job. Thanks to Neil Bernstein for showing us how a real professional photographer works. It was an eye-opening experience to work with you.

A huge thanks to Erin Byron for editing the first drafts. I am sure that Tom also thanks you since it made his job easier. Thank you to Erin Byron, Al Cochrane, Derek Hopkins, and Libby Piper for volunteering your time. It was an absolute treat working with you all. I wish I could make the asana look as easy and elegant as you guys do.

I have been fortunate to have many phenomenal teachers throughout the years. I especially want to thank some of my Feldenkrais teachers whose work, insights, and encouragement have inspired me on my journey. Thanks to Larry Goldfarb for giving me a Feldenkrais lesson in Wisconsin a couple of decades ago. It really changed the way I looked at myself. I also want to thank you, Larry, for all the great writing that you freely share with all of us. Thanks to Jeff Haller for creating workshops and then putting the workshops on DVDs for those of us who can't make it to Seattle. Your insights about movement and strength are second to none. As always, I have to thank my mentor, Yvan Joly. Thanks for always taking time to answer my e-mails and meeting with me when I am in Montreal. Without your guidance, Yvan, I would have been lost a long time ago. All three of you have made an impact on how I look at movement and the development of movement. If you had not freely shared your work with me, I could not have written this book.

To Matt and Michael my "On Your Authority" buddies, chatting with you guys and creating the podcast every other week is a true source of inspiration. Hopefully one day we will even get people to listen to our podcast... Oh well, we have so much fun chatting that we would do it even without an audience!

As always, thanks to all the students I have worked with; you have taught me much more than I have taught you.

To Helena, thanks for putting up with my crazy ideas, traveling with me to Springsteen concerts, putting up with me teaching on weekends way too frequently, and giving me the space to write this book. (I hope I remembered to tell you that I have signed a contract for my next book.)

Last, but not least, thank you to everyone I didn't mention. Thank you for supporting me as I fumble my way through life while creating my own path. As I look back on the path, it looks winding and hilly, and there are dead ends here and there, but it is full of all the many good memories that you all have contributed. Much love to all of you!

introduction

A Story of Collaboration, Innovation, and Perspective

In the study of yoga, it is common to start in one place, only to end up somewhere completely unexpected. The possibilities for learning through yoga are as endless as the practice itself. Ultimately, this book is a story about one of those unexpected journeys. It is the work of two people with similar interests and completely different backgrounds coming together at exactly the right time to influence each other and create a new perspective on yoga therapy practices.

My (Kristen's) curiosity about yoga started in the year 2000. As a lifelong lover of the arts, my first yoga classes fed my natural impulse to explore the varied aspects of consciousness and the human experience. I dove wholeheartedly into the study of yoga, and it changed my life for the better. In 2006, I took a leap of faith and quit my corporate job to participate in an intensive yoga teacher training program. That same year I met and married my husband Bob, who holds a PhD in yoga therapy. My personal immersion into the yoga lifestyle was complete. I began managing certain aspects of the YogaLife Institute, the yoga studio and education center in Pennsylvania that Bob started in 1996, along with editing *Yoga Living* magazine and teaching yoga classes full time.

My yoga journey toward becoming a teacher of teachers evolved at a rapid-fire pace over the next five years. I accumulated thousands of hours of in-class teaching experience and significantly expanded my yoga education, accumulating some 2,500 hours of yoga and anatomy training. Around my fifth year of teaching full time, I experienced a life-changing spinal injury, which took me to physical therapy. The initial work with my physical therapist required that I better understand my movement habits and compensation patterns, and I spent the year completely focused on uncovering old habits and exploring new movement patterns. During that time, I took a break from practicing yoga poses and in doing so began to question some of what I had learned during my intensive training period. As I healed and began to reapproach my yoga practice, I knew that many of the ways that I had been engaging with the yoga poses would have to change. Inspired by the learning that happened in my physical therapy sessions, I began to clearly understand what worked and what didn't, and for my personal learning I augmented my practice by exploring movement practices outside of the field of yoga. Pilates, Feldenkrais, Continuum, Yoga Tune Up Structural Integration, Craniosacral, and Somatic Movement therapies have all revolutionized, invigorated, or supported my personal yoga practice.

My (Staffan's) background growing up as an athlete in Sweden shaped many of my ideas about the body and movement. I have always taken an interest in alternative healing, so it has been natural for me to combine that personal knowledge with my professional experience in the physical therapy world. As a physical therapy practitioner and teacher of physical therapists, I have always found inspiration and insight through studying athletics and somatic movement practices. (Somatic movement practices such as the Feldenkrais Method, Alexander Method, and others emphasize the individual's perceived internal bodily sensations and experiences as a basis for how the person acts in daily activities.) I continue to be fascinated by the experience of movement. Curiosity about creating more awareness through movement eventually led me to become certified in the Feldenkrais method, a training that greatly influenced my perspective on the body and its expressions. Exploring my movements and looking at habits changed the way I experience myself, along with the way I understand culture and society. It also influenced the way that I look at physical therapy.

Over the years I have worked in various settings across the United States, observing how physical therapy is practiced. I have worked with world-class athletes, dancers, musicians, and actors to satisfy my curiosity about how habitual movement can limit performance and expression. For the last eight years, I have taught students at the graduate level in the Physical Therapy program at Nazareth College in New York. My classroom continues to be a laboratory where we explore the intricacies of movement and the human body. A natural evolution of my studies was to explore the field of yoga therapy. As a result, I became involved with the International Association of Yoga Therapists in 2004, and in 2011 joined the Comprehensive Yoga Therapy training program at the YogaLife Institute. A year later, I began collaborating with Kristen and teaching in the program.

The timing of our meeting was fortuitous because we were both ready to explore different perspectives on movement and its relationship to the human experience. During the first years of our collaboration, we got to know one another, asked questions, and shared ideas and resources. Then we reviewed all of the movement practices we had explored over the years and talked about their effects and what the differences and similarities were between them in terms of learning outcomes. What made one method more or less effective, why, and for whom? What does effective really mean in terms of a movement practice? The more we reflected and observed and played with different concepts in our classes and trainings, the more interested we became in how the nervous system evolves by solving movement puzzles. We landed on the concept of habits and created learning structures that use variations of yoga poses to challenge the nervous system. The ability to adapt to new environments and apply learning from yoga practices into our life activities became of particular interest.

During our years of collaboration, we talked a lot about teaching concepts and spent time examining a variety of teaching mechanisms and systems for exploring movement. As educators by nature, we also talked a lot about learning styles, pedagogy, timing, and delivery. At that time we also developed the foundational concepts outlined in this book as we wrote presentations for the Comprehensive Yoga Therapy training program. Of course, the work spilled over into our other classes, workshops, trainings, and sessions with private clients along with our personal practices. When we were lucky, we got to spend whole weekends teaching together, and in this environment, we could observe each other teach and observe students while the other was teaching. After the practices were over, we immediately discussed the students' experiences of the practices. As we continued to teach, observe, listen, and discuss, we could clearly see the efficacy of the principles in the book—**identification**, **differentiation**, and **integration**—reflected back to us in our students' learning outcomes.

The timing was right, and Human Kinetics called Kristen for a proposal just at the point where we had realized that we had enough information to write a book about the perspective we had formed. We were excited about the opportunity to reach folks beyond our classrooms so that they could also experience the benefits of the structures and practices that we had created. The rest of our collaboration story is what you are holding in your hands now. The work has already taken us to new and unexpected places. Who knows where else we will go? For the time being, we are considering it a living thing, and are looking forward to seeing how you will interact with the perspective we are sharing. We are curious about how you will use the structures for practice and what your new levels of integrated awareness will be. It is our hope that the work that you do as a result of reading this book will contribute to the continued enjoyment of all your life's activities.

How to Best Engage With This Book

The purpose of this body of work is to guide you to more deeply understand yourself through applied yoga therapy practice: to identify, differentiate, and integrate the areas of your life that you want to realize more deeply. As you do so, be willing to explore your movement habits in new and creative ways. Open your mind to new experiences and get ready to have fun exploring what is possible in a yoga therapy practice. Once you have a sense of what we are laying out as the framework for your exploration, have fun expanding the framework and connecting the practices into other activities. Whenever you come across a highlighted exploration in the book, do the practices and spend time reflecting on your experience. Understanding the structures that we lay out will be important, but taking the concepts into realized experience will help you make more meaningful and personal connections with what you are learning. This book is organized progressively in three parts.

Part I: Fundamentals of Yoga Therapy

This section introduces the concepts and supporting information about yoga therapy. It will explain the whys and hows of our perspective on yoga therapy practices and illuminate how they can support your active lifestyle. This section starts you on your yoga therapy journey with a variety of thought, movement, and breath explorations. Chapter 1 explores the differences between yoga and yoga therapy. Chapters 2 and 3 introduce you to the movement systems and discuss how to connect the brain to the body, challenge the nervous system, and solve movement puzzles. Here we also introduce the concepts of identification, differentiation, and integration that run throughout the book. Understanding those concepts will help you get the most out of the practices. Chapter 4 builds on that learning and introduces important information and experiences related to breathing, visualization, sensory mastery, and mindfulness. Understanding and applying these practices will enhance the work that you will do later in the book.

Part II: Foundations of Practice

The second part of the book offers insights into creating a practice based on inquiry and curiosity. We start with a look at the creative use of props and then move into exploring the concepts of structural variety, body sensations, cultivating awareness, and the limits of practice. We also explore more experiences with adaptable breathing, meditation, and relaxation. We look at injuries from two perspectives: first, how to prevent injuries in yoga practice and then how to use yoga therapy practices to prevent injuries in other activities. This section sets you up to create an intelligent and sustainable yoga therapy practice for yourself.

Part III: Poses for Lifelong Fitness

The final part of the book builds on everything that you have learned in the previous sections and continues to expand your knowledge base of yoga poses. You will explore the power of intention as you continue to put the principles of identification, differentiation, and integration into practice. You can customize the hundreds of pose variations highlighted in chapters 9 and 10 to support your intentions for your evolving yoga therapy practice. We encourage you to explore and use this part of the book as much and as long as you like—there is enough material to engage you for quite some time. We hope that you come back to this section over and over to adapt and augment your practices as your goals and needs change over the years. The final chapter, chapter 11, gives you more ideas for how to use everything that you have learned in the book to help maintain your active lifestyle. It also introduces new areas for you to focus on and play with as your practice continues to expand and grow.

Happy exploring!

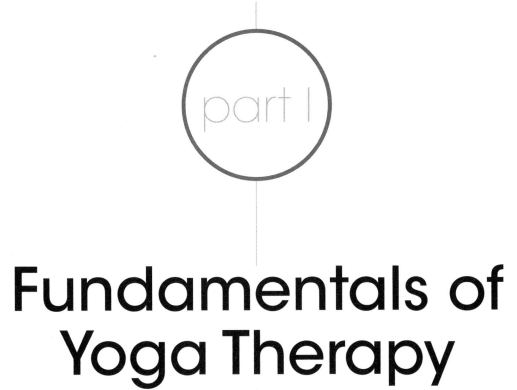

part I

Fundamentals of Yoga Therapy

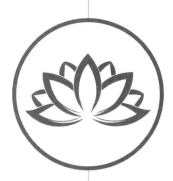

one
What Is Yoga Therapy?

When you think of yoga, what comes to mind? What have you thought, read, or heard about what yoga is—or is not? The answer to this question is as varied as the people who might answer it. Everyone brings with them a unique perspective and history that influences their approach to yoga as an art form or discipline.

There are oversimplifications:

- Yoga is all about stretching.
- Yoga is a religious practice.
- Yoga is a way to keep fit.

There are overreaches:

- Yoga can cure XYZ condition.
- Yoga is good for everyone.
- Yoga is better than therapy.

And there are personal outcomes:

- Yoga helps me deal with my stress.
- Yoga makes me a better person.
- Yoga keeps me balanced.

What's interesting is that within the right context, any of these statements could be considered true, even the oversimplifications and overreaches. Some people consider yoga to be a part of their fitness routine and nothing more. For many people, yoga is part of a rich religious and cultural history. Others see it as a nondogmatic devotional practice. Some folks dabble in all of these things but don't consider themselves to be a "yogi" or "yogini." Anecdotes abound about how yoga helped someone heal a serious health condition, lose weight, manage anxiety, minimize back pain, reduce medications, maximize performance, increase energy, and more.

Chances are you have done some yoga or at least know a few people who have. Perhaps a friend, physical therapist, or chiropractor suggested that you give it a try. Maybe you're a new yoga teacher or seasoned professional continuing your education, hungry for new information that will empower you and your students.

Whether through first- or secondhand experience, you probably have noticed that there are about as many types of yoga as there are flavors of ice cream. Fast-paced classes that leave you needing a good shower and a gallon of water afterward are common offerings at local gyms and studios. Less common, but still available, are classes that gently lull you into a deep state of relaxation that lasts for hours. Esoteric classes focusing on some of the lesser-known aspects of practice such as balancing the chakras, chanting, or meditating also happen in local studios, parks, community centers, clinics, and other venues. If you're lucky, you may have experienced classes that clearly weave a combination of the aforementioned possibilities into a well-rounded practice. While all of these experiences are different and valid, they share a common thread: They fundamentally focus on teaching techniques in a generalized group setting. This is a primary characteristic of what we might call yoga classes or group yoga practices.

Yoga vs. Yoga Therapy

Because you or someone you know may have experienced some kind of profound shift or healing in a group yoga class, it might feel like a leap for us to say that while the outcomes may have been therapeutic, they were not necessarily *yoga therapy*. Yoga therapy may look similar to regular yoga from the outside, but beneath the surface is a discernible difference.

The primary feature of yoga therapy lies in the individualized nature and personalized learning outcomes of the practice. More than a teacher in a group class offering you a skillful adjustment or postural suggestion for the physical practices, it's a practice customized just for you. Yoga therapy takes into consideration the totality of your human experience—the unique combination of your physical body, existing health conditions, individual history, view of the world, disposition, life goals, inter- and intrapersonal relationships, work–life balance, emotional awareness, mental stamina, and sense of spiritual connection. Instead of generalized technique instructions that you must retrofit to your needs, yoga therapy empowers you with support structures from which you create a distinctly personal yoga lifestyle plan.

Yoga Therapy as a Lifestyle Practice

Yoga therapy is intended to be an integrated practice of amplifying, maintaining, and restoring health during the various cycles of life, whether you are already active, looking to become more active, or simply wanting to continue your beloved activities well into your golden years. Using this practice, you can make more conscious and proactive choices to support your health and longevity, which in turn can offer an enhanced experience of daily life.

Yoga therapy participants are encouraged to make healthy choices about work–life balance, nutrition, rest, relationships, movement, and thought patterns. Focusing on lifestyle factors shows promise in the areas of reducing stress, decreasing inflammation in the body, slowing physical and mental degeneration, amplifying the immune response, regulating physiological functions, bringing vitality and energy to the body, managing pain, increasing body awareness, and improving musculoskeletal function. In this way, yoga therapy supports the entire person—body, energy, senses, intellect, and spirit—in the quest to stay vital and active.

Yoga therapy offers foundational lifestyle guidance from traditional yogic texts, most notably the *Yoga Sutras of Patanjali*, the *Upanishads*, *Hatha Yoga Pradipika*, and the *Bhagavad Gita*. This vastly rich tradition is now incorporated into modern health care and is studied by a diverse group of scientists and medical practitioners. Scientists are applying their own definitions and understanding of how yoga works to relieve a myriad of psychological and physical ailments. These coalesced resources provide us with scientific insights, offering general guidelines for active, healthy living. Practices include movement, breathing exercises, mental techniques, lifestyle education, and philosophies on personal growth that are intended to bring physical and psychological processes into balance.

Growing Evidence Base

We live in exciting times when the more traditional practices of yoga are meeting the needs of modern society and are included in cutting-edge scientific research. Although this kind of study offers amazing new insights into how the ancient practices work as a healing discipline, it also has pitfalls. It is challenging to quantify something as vast and holistic as yoga therapy. When the entirety of the human experience is taken into consideration, where does a researcher start? Is it even possible to pinpoint where and how the healing happens? Is it the poses, breathing exercises, changes in attitude, reduction of stress, improvement in sleep, meditation practices, better diet, or the increased sense of spiritual connection that brought about changes? It's tempting to point to one thing and say, "That's it; that is what healed me" but often that is not the case with the holistic model. One change begets another, and it is often the connections we make between things that are at the core of our most powerful healing experiences.

As yoga therapists, we want to be careful about fitting into the reductionist scientific model, while remaining open to integrating the insights and understandings that come out of scientific studies. Many smart, dedicated people in the field of yoga therapy are working to better quantify how the practices work. The applications that are coming out of the scientific studies are paving the way for yoga therapy to be accepted into the mainstream health care system, which is important for the field to progress. But we need to remain aware that trying to retrofit the vastness of yoga therapy into the healthcare model, or reducing yoga therapy to a set of standardized techniques, has the potential to greatly reduce its usefulness.

This requires that practitioners in the field of yoga therapy cooperate with and learn from research, but without being beholden to the scientific model. We need to look at how the research fits into the bigger picture so that we can refine our scientific understanding of how yoga therapy works and at the same time keep the holistic perspective intact. We think of this as an evolving dialogue between the traditional mind–body orientation of yoga practices and the established fields of medicine, psychology, anatomy, biomechanics, biology, kinesiology, and neuroscience. It is possible that we will be able to pinpoint the exact mechanism of action in some cases, but in others we won't. Not knowing exactly how something works shouldn't deter us from using it if it does. This living in and exploring unquantifiable territory can be uncomfortable, but in many ways it is the essence of yoga itself.

Some of the most promising research supporting the use of yoga therapy is coming out of the field of neuroscience. This book will use the nervous system as a guide for practice, offering structures to cultivate deeper levels of awareness, sensitivity, and responsiveness. Practicing from the perspective of the nervous system offers a template from which you can make more informed choices that carry over into optimal functioning in daily life. It will also increase the amount of pleasure you take from all of your activities.

Healing: Holistic Model vs. Medical Model

When we talk about achieving optimal health through yoga therapy, one of the most interesting considerations is shifting from a medical model to a holistic model of treatment. A medical model assumes a subject–object relationship between the health care provider and client. This means that the provider (subject) is expected to effect some kind of change in the patient or client (object). The basic expectation is that this change will be achieved through assessment, diagnosis, and some kind of intervention such as drugs, surgery, or therapy. The patient is deemed a passive recipient of treatment rather than a proactive participant in his or her own healing process.

Tell me, and I'll forget. Show me, and I may not remember. Involve me, and I will understand.

—Author unknown

It's important to note that many medical practitioners do not necessarily want to function in this way. While they may encourage their patients to take more responsibility for their health, it is not within their professional scope to provide the supporting structures from which those changes can happen. Patients may leave the doctor's office with a recommendation to reduce their stress, improve their diet, or increase their exercise but have no idea how to actually go about it. While the medical practitioners can inform their patients that health is connected to implementing some course of action, the subject–object model they are working under doesn't allow them to follow up on the implementation of their recommendations. It is up to patients to create or seek other support from which lifestyle changes can be implemented.

The subject–object model has real advantages when dealing with acute cases that need diagnostic support and solutions. In crucial life-and-death scenarios such as an appendix that is about to burst, a serious accident, or emergency surgery, patients cannot proactively respond to what is happening in the moment. However, if they use yoga therapy lifestyle principles to take care of themselves before the acute distress, they have set the stage for an improved immune response and expedited recovery.

The subject–object model has been less successful in dealing with lifestyle diseases such as type 2 diabetes, some types of cancer and heart disease, arthritis, osteoporosis, hypertension, and common digestive disorders. It might be convenient for patients to let their doctors treat the symptoms of a lifestyle disease. But it is a false convenience because although these interventions might be helpful at the onset of symptoms, they typically do not resolve the root causes. When we couple the tendency to treat the symptoms instead of the cause with the fact that many common medications have side effects that are just as bad as—and sometimes worse than—the original complaints, patients become trapped in a cycle of disempowerment and unnecessary suffering. This is where the holistic model of yoga therapy can be an invaluable companion to current health care practices. Yoga therapy is not a replacement for modern medicine or psychological counseling. Instead, it helps patients establish healthy patterns and lifestyle choices that support the work they are already doing with their doctor, psychologist, physical therapist, chiropractor, nutritionist, or other health care provider.

As the name implies, the holistic model emphasizes the importance of the whole human being and exploring the interdependence of its parts. Yoga therapy designates the different aspects of human experience into five layers of reality that are known as the koshas. They progress from the gross (that which is more tangible) to subtle (less tangible) in this order: physical, energetic, emotional, intellectual, and spiritual.

In addition to the holistic perspective, a multitude of yoga therapy practices can be used to keep the active person active. These include movement explorations, yoga poses, breathing lessons, exercises to increase mental clarity, and other processes that support personal growth and evolution.

Yoga Therapy as a Call to Personal Action

Traditional yoga practices offer a set of guidelines for fulfilling one's potential, known as self-realization. People who choose to fully engage in this process use these structures as a mechanism for deeper levels of self-understanding. It starts with learning how to slow down and be less reactive and more capable of paying attention to what is happening in the present moment. This awareness allows them to identify and eventually implement yoga practices that will help forge healthy mind–body connections.

As you gain new layers of self-awareness and understanding, yoga also offers tools to deconstruct your belief systems, see where your habits hurt or help, and understand the different yet interconnected layers of your reality. Yoga teaches that although you might not always be able to control the external environment, you do have a choice to differentiate your internal environment from your external one and with it, an opportunity to understand your habitual reactions to external stimulus. Instead of looking outside for external cues for how to behave, you can start to look within yourself for the power to make less reactionary and more conscious choices.

The perspectives on yoga therapy presented in this book are designed to support your active life. It offers a multitude of tools to help increase your awareness of how you think, feel, move, and act so that you can begin, get back to, or continue to enjoy the activities you love. You will learn how to integrate old and new habits so that you can choose optimal movements from a whole-person response, rather than simply reacting to what is happening outside of you. The book is full of tools to help you to make proactive choices for your health and longevity.

Movement: A Key to Health and Longevity

Every activity that you do (or don't do) affects your body and brain in some way. The choices that you make about your movement practices, diet, sleep habits, preventive health care, work–life balance, emotional health, relationships, and spirituality all have tremendous impact on your health and longevity.

Life is a cycle of activity and rest. When you are lucky, activity and rest flow together seamlessly, creating a sense of harmony and balance. It is a glorious day indeed when even the most mundane activity is imbued with a sense of purpose: each action executed with some combination of intention, mindfulness, energetic awareness, emotional intelligence, and physical vigor. Too little or too much activity can bring you out of balance, and you can feel fatigued, fragmented, overwhelmed,

[handwritten margin note:] yoga helps us to develop new levels of self awareness making it possible to slowly create change

[handwritten margin note:] It's in your choices what you decide is just your responsibility

or stressed. When out of balance or operating on autopilot, you end up getting less pleasure from life in general.

Activity often enriches our life experiences. The *World Sports Encyclopedia* estimates that there are at least 8,000 indigenous sports and sporting games. With so many incredible sport and game options, it can be difficult to choose which to pursue. Beyond sports and games, are other activities that we associate with a well-lived life—taking walks, engaging with friends, playing with kids, traveling to new places, cooking tasty food, or pursuing creative activities such as painting, crafting, constructing or deconstructing, making music or dancing to its beat. It can be difficult to find the time for all of the activities we would like to have in our life.

> *Movement is life. Life is a process. Improve the quality of the process and you improve the quality of life itself.*
>
> —Moshe Feldenkrais, founder of the Feldenkrais Method (R) and Awareness Through Movement (R)

Some activities are more alluring than others. What you find to be a pleasant activity (or not) depends on your natural gifts, disposition, upbringing, energy levels, attitudes toward life, and beliefs about work and effort. Of course, activities and the necessary balance of rest can vary greatly from person to person. Factors to consider include phase of life, physical condition, location, occupation, and most important, healthy energy levels.

If you have picked up this book, chances are you are motivated to do some of these things:

- Be more proactive and self-reliant about your health
- Maintain or upgrade your current activity levels
- Harness your mental focus
- Manage your stress
- Boost your energy levels
- Effect change through a personalized yoga therapy practice
- "Prehabilitate" your body so that you can continue to enjoy the activities you love, injury free as you age.
- Rehabilitate your body from illness or injury so that you can get back to doing the activities you love
- Enhance performance of your life activities
- Experience more enjoyment from your life activities

The awareness that is born out of a personalized yoga therapy plan can touch on one or all of these areas; the potential really is that vast. And while the broad and comprehensive nature of yoga therapy is not the primary focus of this book, you can certainly pay attention to how introducing its mind–body movement practices affects these other aspects of your life. When you invite changes to the body, it is inevitable that new awareness will arise and that you will make related shifts in the mind and spirit as a result.

Why Yoga Therapy in the Modern Age?

It's no secret that technology is changing our bodies and brains. If you were born before the 1970s and can remember a time when you didn't have a smart phone, laptop, tablet, or flat screen as part of your daily routine, you have probably already sensed these changes in yourself and seen them in those around you. There have been profound changes in the way we live and communicate. Technology and convenience have changed everything: how we socialize, how we process information, how we feel, how we eat, how we sleep, and how we see the world.

The inherent imbalance in activity for the modern human is that while we are moving our bodies less, our minds are taking in more information than ever. Take a moment to consider the implications of that statement. The body and brain are good at adapting and sorting, but what have we lost during this particular evolution? Although many scientists, anthropologists, doctors, physical therapists, educators, nutritionists, yoga therapists, and other smart people are asking this question and even creating solutions, it might take time before we completely comprehend what the impact of living in the technological age means for modern human beings, along with our continued evolution.

One of the most common challenges for the modern human is remaining connected to the body and its processes. Being out of touch with the body results in a decreased ability to execute basic healthy movement patterns. The simple acts of squatting, crawling, rolling, rotating, bending, kneeling, balancing, standing, and walking on varied surfaces have tremendous value for all of the systems of the body. Conscious movement can affect more aspects of our health than we previously thought possible—muscles, bones, organs, glands, and nerves can be positively affected—all the way down to a cellular level by turning on or off certain patterns of longevity. It's not just the amount of sitting that affects our lives (which is a lot), but also the lack of variety in our daily movements compared to that of our ancestors. That lack of variety is changing our brains, altering our body composition, impeding developmental patterns, and shortening life spans.

Active people who do yoga and exercise regularly are still at risk for this diminished capacity. Going to the gym, playing a sport, hiking, or hitting a yoga class a couple of times a week won't undo the damage that 40 to 60 hours per week of sitting might cause. Couple that with the fact that many people are out of touch with their bodies as they perform repetitive exercises, and we have a recipe for loss of function and injury. The "no pain, no gain" mentality that is so prevalent in modern exercise culture doesn't help either. It is likely that many people who exercise are duplicating their inefficient or unrefined movement patterns of daily life in their exercise sessions, only faster and with more vigor.

Although many of the movements that are included in this book could be considered exercise, we suggest that you think of them more as daily actions to challenge your nervous system and give your body and brain new forms of input. Small actions performed with awareness throughout the day can effect big changes in the body and mind.

Individualism and Inquiry

In a world that continually conspires to draw your attention outward, seeking external input and approval, the act of personal inquiry can fly in the face of cultural norms. Although it may be uncomfortable at times, becoming aware and making fully conscious life choices offers you the potential to live and act based on internal awareness—at peace with yourself regardless of what is happening in the external world.

One of the many reasons for the growing popularity of yoga therapy is that it offers a broad umbrella of concepts, techniques, and practices from which you can inquire into your internal sense of self. You get to choose the level and type of awareness that you want to develop, and the yoga therapist acts as a professional guide along the path.

It is nothing short of a miracle that modern methods of instruction have not yet entirely strangled the holy curiosity of inquiry.

—Albert Einstein

Yoga therapy allows you to explore yourself more deeply and empowers you to be a more proactive participant in how you experience life. You are enlivened by your engagement with a deeper sense of self. The nervous system helps you gain more self-understanding. When you are aware of your internal cues and use them to be more responsive to the needs of the nervous system in various environments, the brain can change size and shape with new input (neuroplasticity). This in turn makes you even more responsive, sensitive, and resilient as you learn.

As you process the information related to yoga practices, it is important to recognize that everyone is unique and will respond differently based on previous conditioning, beliefs, and intentions for practice. The health and fitness culture has a tendency to make the individual experience a universal one: This is how *I* improved my strength, so you should do it the same way too. Another proclivity is for people to speak in absolutes. Here are the most common:

- This is the correct way to do it.
- You're going about it all wrong.
- Do this, not that.

This tendency to speak in absolutes or authoritarian tones was established long ago, and we could probably write an entire book on the psychological, societal, religious, and political reasons for why this style of communication has become so prevalent in modern yoga culture. But that is not the focus of this book, so suffice it to say that this tendency exists, and it can leave people feeling confused or disempowered at some point during their journey toward a healthy, active lifestyle.

In the yoga world, there's no shortage of teachers who will tell what you *must* or *have to* do for your yoga practice to be authentic, correct, in proper alignment, or whatever terms of authority they might use. There's even a nickname in our culture for them: the yoga police. You might find them patrolling at gyms, studios, retreat centers, or most frequently in the comments section of social media feeds and blogs.

You will notice that the tone of this book is distinctly different from that of the yoga police. One of the cornerstones of our unique approach is a focus on personal inquiry. Rather than telling you what is right or wrong, we prefer to encourage you to notice, sense, feel, perceive, breathe, and respond to the practices as they unfold. The act of paying attention and inquiring is an art unto itself. In the face of a world that offers endless opportunities for distraction, it is no small undertaking. For this reason, we encourage you to be compassionate and patient with yourself as you hone your attention skills.

And while we honor the inquiry as much as finding answers where possible, we are also educators and experts in our fields. By nature, we have spent many years testing our hypotheses, garnering feedback from peers and students, and refining our processes. Our work has led us to eschew dogma and shudder at absolutes.

Subsequently, our programs are engineered to encourage students to explore the principles of yoga therapy in a way that is highly personal and immediately meaningful.

We start with the assumption that there is nothing wrong with you and that you are already doing the best that you can with the information you've been given. Our job as educators is to organize meaningful structures through which you can explore your intentions and actions and create an environment in which transformation can happen. Simply put, we are here to offer guidance that allows you to explore yoga therapy. We give you history, philosophy, and practices to connect the traditional to the needs of the modern day so you can better sense what yoga therapy might mean to you in the here and now. We offer a clear path that allows for growth and exploration. Rather than boxing you into any one perspective, our goal is that you use this book to start or continue your journey into yoga therapy. Then we encourage you to augment that in any way that makes it more relevant to your goals for an active lifestyle.

As you become a student of your body and mind and fine-tune your discernment skills, self-awareness will morph into self-empowerment. You will move forward in your yoga therapy practices with confidence based on your own developing inquiry. Let's begin!

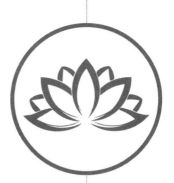

two

Training Movements

This chapter focuses on the body's movement system. It includes a brief overview of relevant anatomy, the nervous system, and how the brain ties it all together in a chosen activity, resulting in greater efficiency and movement quality. We break down the stages of learning new movements and provide simple tips for how to engage this learning and why it is important. We offer examples and movement explorations to highlight how yoga therapy helps you work more skillfully with the nervous system in order to create more options in all of life's activities.

Overview of the Movement System

We move all the time. Many of our movements may be unsound, habitual, and automatic, but they are still movements. We even move in our sleep. What is the system that guides and informs those movements? What we believe about the movement system has not changed in roughly 100 years. What has changed is our view of how much each component of the movement system contributes to the entire action. The movement system has three fundamental parts:

1. Muscles (muscles, tendons, fascia)
2. Skeleton (bones, joints, ligaments)
3. Nervous system (central nervous system, peripheral nervous system)

Here is how movement occurs: The muscles connect to the bones through tendons, the bones connect to each other by ligaments, and the nervous system tells the muscles to fire, which pulls the tendons so the bones move. Simple, right? Well, it appears that movement is not that simple.

As we improve our ability to look into the body in noninvasive ways, we also improve our understanding of movement. Our view of the interactions between components of the movement system has changed. While we still consider the three fundamental components to be the same—muscles, skeleton, nervous system—we now know that many internal and external factors influence our movements and especially the way the nervous system works.

Lifestyle factors that affect the nervous system, such as sadness, nutrition, anxiety, sleepiness, anger, motivation, and other stressors, also alter the way we move. We might move faster, slower, more carefully, or more aggressively based on the context of our situation. The signals the nervous system receives from the internal and external environments and the signals it sends out affect our movements much more than previously believed.

This new view about how the movement system's parts interact is more difficult to comprehend because it is more complicated to visualize. It is easy to picture the muscles moving the skeleton based on a message the brain sent to the muscles through the nerves. It is more difficult to imagine that the context we are in actually changes the impulses the nervous system sends to the muscles. The good news is that the nervous system is more or less ready to act in a variety of those internal and external contexts even though countless influences on the nervous system affect each action. It is difficult to fathom the complexities that go into creating movement. The nervous system's job is to solve the puzzle of the context and how to conduct the most effective, efficient movement in that situation.

If the nervous system cannot find a solution to a movement puzzle or select the appropriate action in a certain context, the result might be pain or an unconscious avoidance of that particular movement. The more movements you avoid, the more you avoid living a fulfilling, active life.

Even when you think you have performed an action in the same way as before, the nervous system may activate muscles in a different way based on the context you are in. We take the viewpoint in this book that movement is largely influenced and governed by the nervous system. Thus, to stay active throughout life, you must not only work the muscles, but also make sure your nervous system is fit and ready to learn. We look at yoga therapy as a form of somatic education (learning through the living body) and at yoga poses (known as asanas in the yoga community) as a way to teach the nervous system to solve movement puzzles.

Yoga therapy can make you more aware of changes in the nervous system and other aspects of the movement system. When you use yoga therapy, you become more sensitive to movement—how it changes based on your context and habits and how you can create more options. By bringing awareness to the movement system, activities become more enjoyable, you perform them with less effort, and you are able to consciously adjust the way you perform the activity based on the current context.

To ensure these benefits of yoga therapy, the following is essential:

- Pay attention to the movements and actions.
- Practice a variety of yoga asanas.
- Do the asanas in a variety of ways.

We now know that variety is what maintains the health of the movement system and will keep you active throughout life. Variety keeps the nervous system healthy and happy. Performing yoga asanas the same way day in and day out is no better than performing any unvaried movement. Remember that the nervous system is a puzzle solver, and if it doesn't have a problem to solve it becomes "lazy." Varying your movements creates challenges for the nervous system. When the nervous system solves the movement puzzle, you can observe changes not only in movement patterns, but also in your behavior! A changed movement or behavior pattern is a sure sign of learning in the movement system. Before we delve further into what we mean by learning in the movement system, let's look a little deeper into the components of the movement system.

Bones, Muscles, and Fascia

The musculoskeletal system is made up of the skeleton, muscles, ligaments, tendons, and fascia. A human skeleton consists of 206 bones and there are approximately 650 muscles. Traditionally, muscles and bones have received the most attention in the musculoskeletal part of the movement system (figure 2.1). It is easy to understand why. We can see muscles under our skin and we can feel the bones of the skeleton in several places on our body. When scientists initially dissected cadavers, they divided the body where it seemed to make sense: muscles where they attached to bones by tendons and bones where they met at joints. They pulled at the muscles

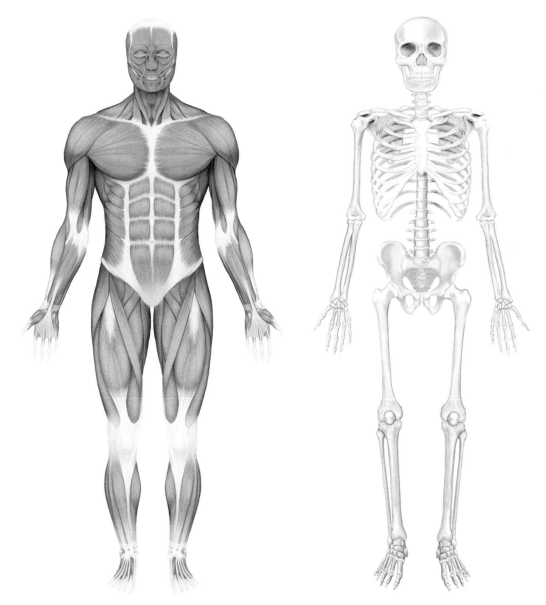

Figure 2.1   The muscles and bones of the musculoskeletal system.

and saw that the pull from the muscles generated specific movements of the bones. Thus, the division into muscles and bones made sense and was easy to do.

Most cadavers used for science were, and still are, older cadavers that had been preserved. What is not easily visible or missing from preserved cadavers is the fascia, the thin sheath of fibrous tissue enclosing muscles and other organs and creating a continuous whole of the body. Starting in the 1950s and up to the present day, brilliant people such as Ida Rolf, Tom Myers, and Robert Schleip saw patterns in the fascia and developed models for how it might influence the patterns of the body. Ida Rolf developed Rolfing as a method of working with the fascia, Tom Myers developed his Anatomy Trains system, and Robert Schleip started researching the role of fascia in the movement system. But even before the recent research into the fascia, a medical doctor from Prague named Vladimir Janda saw common patterns in people's bodies.

Janda (1968), a rehabilitation physician from the Czech Republic, saw rehabilitation through the lens of the sensorimotor system. He considered many of the common rehabilitation issues to be a matter of faulty motor control, not isolated muscle weakness or tightness. Instead of doing what was common at the time and focusing on the first two components of the movement system—muscles and bones—he placed more emphasis on the nervous system.

Janda worked with the nervous system via motor control and functional stability. He took a global view of movement dysfunction and stated that dysfunction in any of the three components of the movement system would show up not only at a local level, but also at a global level throughout the organism. He also looked at how anatomy and kinesiology were integrated throughout a person and called that "functional anatomy." From there, Janda developed an understanding of how dysfunctions in the movement system tended to happen in certain patterns.

Janda (1987) divided the muscles into groups that were considered either hyperactive (overactive) or hypoactive (underactive). From the idea of hyper- and hypoactive muscles, Janda (1987) (1988) developed the theory of the upper and lower crossed syndromes. Upper crossed syndrome (UCS) can be characterized as the typical forward-head and rounded-shoulder posture that is so common (figure 2.2), especially among people in the modern world who have desk jobs and are living sedentary lifestyles. Lower crossed syndrome (LCS) includes short hip flexors and a rounded low back (figure 2.3).

In Janda's (1987) opinion, the cause of postural syndromes is alterations in motor control leading to faulty muscle firing patterns. Hyperactive muscles fire too easily and are short and tight, while the hypoactive muscles are inhibited—less readily activated with movements—and weak. This leads the weak muscles to atrophy and the tight muscles to shorten even more. Slow-twitch muscles, which tend to be used in endurance activities (in this case proper posture or holding a strong asana for a long time) tend to tighten, and fast-twitch muscles, which are suited for fast bursts of power (such as standing up or doing flow yoga), tend to weaken. Janda made rehabilitation professionals realize that more was needed than just stretching the tight, slow-twitch muscles and strengthening the weak, fast-twitch muscles in isolation. Instead, Janda viewed dysfunction as a condition of the entire movement system, including the nervous system. As we continue to learn, the view of the movement system as a whole has taken on increased importance and that view includes the fascia.

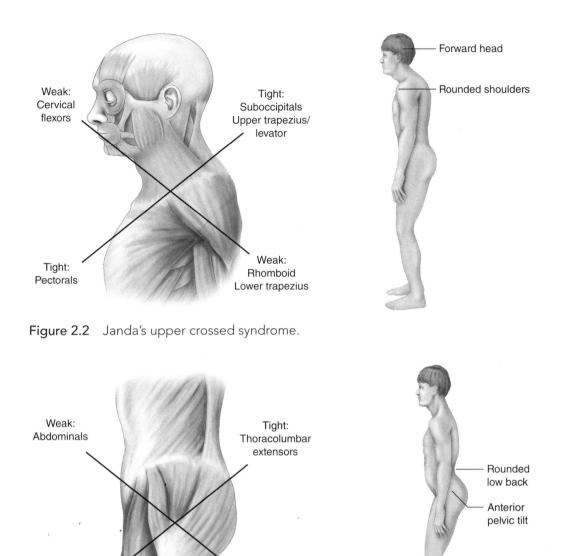

Figure 2.2 Janda's upper crossed syndrome.

Figure 2.3 Janda's lower crossed syndrome.

Fascia connects the structures of the body into a seamless whole (figure 2.4). Instead of dividing the body into specific muscles, tendons, and bones, we now know that the fascia allows the muscles to blend into the tendons, and the tendons to blend into bones. The fascia connects the structures of the body and creates wholeness.

Remember that fascia is connective tissue that envelops the structures of the body. Visceral fascia surrounds the internal organs. More important for the movement system is how the fascia envelops the muscles. Layers of fascia surround not only each muscle, but also each muscle bundle and muscle fiber. At the end of the muscle, fascia then blends into tendon, which then blends into bone.

Fascia is not a new concept or newly discovered type of tissue. Fascia is a structure that has been neglected for a long time, or at least its function has been neglected. When scientists divided the body into distinct parts and named muscles, bones, tendons, and other structures, categorizing the fascia was difficult because it could not be divided into obvious parts. Fascia is found throughout the body and historically was considered a part of something else or a wrapping of the muscles. Often the fascia was not considered worthy of study, so it was removed from cadavers.

That view is changing rapidly. Today worldwide fascia conferences present and explore more and more theories about the function and importance of fascia. The whole musculoskeletal system is connected through the fascia.

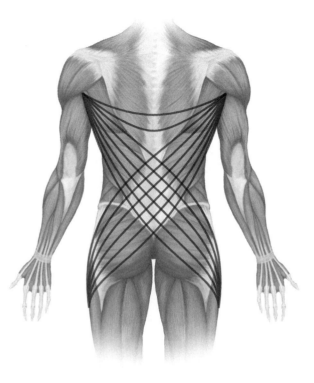

Figure 2.4 Fascia is connective tissue integrated throughout the body.

When you do yoga asanas with varied, nonhabitual movements, you are really engaging the fascial system much more effectively than in regular straight-line stretching.

Myers, with his Anatomy Trains concept, has had a significant impact on how body workers, yoga teachers, movement teachers, and rehabilitation personnel think of fascia. Myers and others have made professionals think of fascia as more than just a wrapping. He looked at how muscles and bones connect through the fascia and came up with the idea of fascial lines. Rather than dividing the body into distinct categories of muscles and bones, he looked at how the muscles and bones were connected in vertical integration throughout the body. Myers identified seven main fascial lines in the body.

Determining the seven fascial lines required Myers to look at the body in terms of connected layers instead of dividing it in a traditional anatomical way. Gil Hedley also looked at the body in this manner and has published wonderful videos of this view. Myers, Hedley, and other integrative experts look at how the body functions as a whole. Some theories hold that fascia functions as a sensory organ and energetic conduit, that it supports organs and stores water, and that it is a transmitter of force. Many other theories exist on the function of fascia. With research expanding rapidly, we see that we are likely early in the process of understanding fascia's complete role. The nervous system is better understood than the fascial system. However, we have only recently become aware of how much the nervous system affects the entire movement system.

Nervous System

The more we learn about the nervous system, the more we realize how much it influences our actions and behavior. Puzzle solving is one of its main roles in movement. It may be solving how to avoid pain, learn a new movement, or improve a habitual pattern. This section's emphasis is on the impact of the nervous system on the whole human being and talks about the central and peripheral nervous systems, as well as the sympathetic and parasympathetic branches of the autonomic nervous system.

The nervous system is divided into the central nervous system (CNS) and peripheral nervous system (PNS) (figure 2.5). The CNS consists of the brain and spinal cord, while the PNS consists of the nerves and ganglia (nerve bundles) that are outside the CNS. To simplify, we can say that the CNS receives and integrates information from the PNS and then decides what to do with that information.

The PNS sends information to the CNS. The CNS integrates that information and creates an appropriate response. This response is based on personal considerations

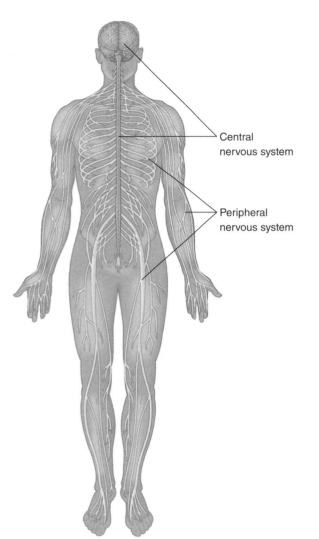

Figure 2.5 The central nervous system and peripheral nervous system.

beyond the information from the PNS, such as the person's experiences in similar situations, the context of the information, and the perceived emergency of the situation. The CNS response is usually outside of a person's awareness and sometimes goes haywire, but we have to remember that the CNS creates the best response it can based on the information it has and the available resources.

Once the CNS creates the appropriate response, the PNS carries out the suggested action and then sends back information about whether the problem was solved. Based on that data, new suggestions for actions are sent from the CNS to the PNS. Information is constantly exchanged between them.

Our own awareness of the nervous system input and output empowers its problem-solving process. We can interrupt the automatic response, thereby delaying it so we can choose to carry it out or not. Many of the CNS responses are habitual responses and do not offer us a variety of movement, behavior, or even mood. Through awareness, if we prefer, we can come up with more appropriate movement solutions to fit our current context. Awareness is key to choosing effectively.

When you practice yoga with awareness, you increase your ability to recognize some of your habitual responses and may notice that they are not optimal for the activities you want to perform. These might be automatic responses regarding perceived or expected pain, reactions to certain motions, or habitual movements that get in the way of performing activities efficiently. Performing yoga asanas with awareness can help you identify which automatic responses are useful and which are not, stop habitual movement, teach the nervous system a more efficient movement solution, and then create more optimal responses. Using awareness to interrupt automatic responses sounds like a simple thing, but it might not be as easy as it sounds.

The tricky thing about interrupting automatic responses is that they have created "tracks" in our brains. There is truth to the saying, "Neurons that fire together, wire together." When we are born few "tracks" have been laid down in our neurons, but there are lots of neurons and connections and many more neurons just waiting to strengthen their connections. As we age, we strengthen connections between neurons that connect frequently and weaken connections between neurons that don't. You could say we "prune the neuron tree" inside the brain to become more organized.

The CNS responses become ever more orderly, and by adulthood we may lose the flexibility to solve movement puzzles in anything other than our habitual ways. Neurons that fire together, wire together. The neurons follow their habitual tracks. Our movement options become increasingly narrow. Some habitual movement is healthy. For example, we take comfort in a morning routine—not having to figuring out how to get out of bed, get dressed, exercise, fix breakfast. However, if all movements were habitual, we would stop challenging the nervous system. When the CNS falls into overly organized, habitual patterns, we stop growing. This makes us less able to adapt and less likely to explore and enjoy new situations.

How adaptable are you? The sitting to standing movement exploration will clue you into your own habitual movement patterns and give you an idea of how to teach the nervous system to solve movement puzzles.

During this exercise, you may find that some combinations make it more difficult to come to standing than others. Did you notice a slight hesitation sometimes? Maybe you couldn't do it at all. Those glitches are the nervous system figuring out a nonhabitual solution to a movement problem. The more habitual your movements are and the longer those habits have been present, the longer the nervous system has to "think" about how to solve a new way of moving.

Although these were simple movement puzzles, this type of exploration can also be applied to other movements. Can you walk, perform your favorite exercise, or stretch in a nonhabitual way? Later in this book, we give you ideas for how to perform asanas in habitual and nonhabitual ways. Give your nervous system the chance to solve problems! You will stay active longer and have more fun if your nervous system is flexible.

Please note that yoga (and other conscious movement practices) do not remove habitual movement options. Yoga brings awareness to how you move and act. By increasing your awareness through yoga therapy, you can choose movements that make your activities more enjoyable, decrease your likelihood of injury during the activities, and allow you to stay active as long as you choose. To find awareness

EXPLORATION
Sitting to Standing

1 Sit in a chair. Stand up from the seated position. How did you go from sitting to standing? Were you aware of how you got up to standing? Were your feet right next to each other, or was one in front of the other?

2 Sit down again. Move the right foot in front of the left and stand up. Sit down. Move the left foot in front of the right and stand up.

3 Consider whether you sensed a difference between these three methods? Was it easier to come to standing one way or the other?

4 Repeat steps 1 through 3 and notice your head. Did you look up or down as you stood up? Can you change the position of your head and stand up? Did that make it easier or more difficult?

5 Sit down, stand up, turn, and take a step to the right. Now do the same thing but turn and take a step to the left. Can you do that again but play with the position of the feet?

of both your internal body signals and external influences, you must find a certain amount of silence and rest in the nervous system. Chapter 1 talked about balance in life; you also need balance in the nervous system.

Many, if not most, people in the Western world live busy lives: work, family, and the constant pull of checking e-mail, text messages, phone, Facebook, and who knows what else. We are constantly "on." Even on vacation, many people carry their smartphone to stay connected. All this connectedness can create an imbalance in the autonomic nervous system.

The autonomic nervous system (ANS) is a part of the peripheral nervous system. The ANS influences the visceral organs and is important in regulating heart rate, respiratory rate, digestion, and many other internal functions. The ANS is divided into the sympathetic and parasympathetic nervous systems. The sympathetic nervous system (SNS) is known as the "fight, flight, or freeze" part of the ANS, while the parasympathetic nervous system (PNS) is the "rest and digest" mode, which is said to have a dampening effect on the SNS. The SNS is activated during periods of stress—the heart rate increases; peristalsis (movement of the digestive tract and other hollow organs) decreases; blood flow to the heart, lungs, and CNS increases. The body is getting ready for action to fight or flee its way out of danger or to freeze to avoid it. This makes sense in a crisis, but is not meant to be chronic.

It is not healthy to be SNS driven for too long because it is a catabolic state that breaks down the body. If the SNS is in command for a long time, the body never has a chance to heal and recharge. The PNS, on the other hand, slows the heart and respiratory rates, allows peristalsis, improves absorption of nutrients, and lowers blood pressure. PNS activation has an anabolic effect on the body. It rejuvenates and rebuilds.

SNS and PNS can also have an effect on learning new movements and activities. When we are stressed we don't learn new movements or facts as easily. In fact, we tend to revert back to our default way of performing activities. With the SNS more active during stress, we need to activate the PNS for optimum learning conditions. How do we activate the PNS? One of the best ways is by slowing down and paying attention to the breath.

The breath is one of the few autonomic functions under our conscious control. Yoga therapy places a lot of emphasis on the breath. Coordinating the breath with movements is a common aspect of all styles of yoga. You could say that without this coordination between breath and movement, yoga is just regular exercise. Conversely, you might also say that any movement coordinated with the breath is yoga. The following movement exploration helps you explore your breath–movement connection.

EXPLORATION
Breath–Movement

❶ While standing, raise your arms out to the sides (*a*) and up overhead (*b*). What did you notice?

❷ Do the same thing, but now coordinate the lifting of your arms with the in-breath, and the lowering of the arms with the out-breath. Did you feel a difference?

❸ Repeat the movement, but reverse the breathing. Lift the arms while breathing out and lower them while breathing in. For most people, this feels odd. It is as if the body were working against itself. In yoga we tend to coordinate the lifting of the arms with the in-breath and the lowering of the arms with the out-breath. That is the more natural way to do this movement. Sometimes you may give your nervous system a puzzle and lift your arms on the out-breath and lower them on the in-breath.

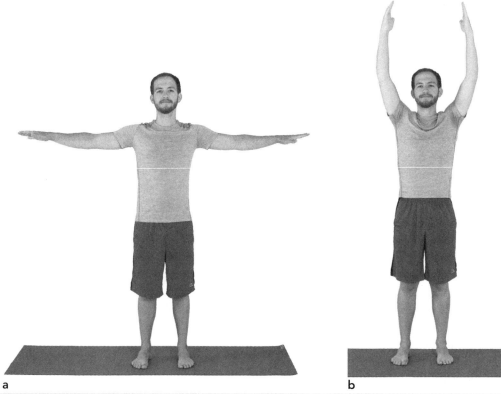

a

b

Later in this chapter, we will look at the importance of p
slowly for optimum motor learning to occur. For now, kı
and slow movement can activate the PNS and put you in
and healing can occur.

The nervous system plays a key role in the movement syste
nal and external information and coming up with the best m
puzzle at hand. Varying and learning new movements happen
dampened and the PNS is more active, in other words, when y
aware. Yoga therapy gives you the tools to consciously bring rela
to your movements. Once you are able to vary your movements
refine them. The following section discusses the process and sigi
vating efficient movement.

Efficient Movement: What It Is and How It Benefits Us

Efficient movement is what everyone wants. But what is it and how is efficient movement different from effective movement? First, let's make clear that we are all moving with the maximum efficiency our nervous system allows. That is, we do our best with the resources we are aware of—not necessarily the resources that we have.

The nervous system solves the problem of doing something, or moving toward or away from something, in the most efficient way it can. To accomplish a task in the most efficient way possible, the puzzle-solving machine of the nervous system figures out the best method based on the resources available, the context the task has to be completed in, and several other factors. If you complete the task, you could say it was performed effectively. This is not the same as being efficient. Effective just means that you produced the intended result, while efficient means that you completed the task with little wasted time or effort. That is a big difference.

For example, let's observe a baby learning to walk. She sees something and wants to reach it. The baby will learn to move efficiently enough to effectively reach the object. If she can crawl to the object there is no need to learn to walk; she will just keep crawling to effectively accomplish the task. If the baby wants to increase how quickly she can reach the object, she will have to figure out a way to do it faster. She tries standing up and walking toward the object. Initially, she does so by holding onto something, but eventually she needs to get to something that is in the middle of the floor where there is nothing to hold onto. It might take a while, but through trial and error and many falls, eventually the baby learns to walk without falling. She can reach the object in the middle of the floor faster and more efficiently by walking than crawling. More-challenging tasks force the nervous system to figure out more efficient ways to move. It may be just as effective to crawl to reach the object, but it is not as fast or efficient!

Another example might be an active adult who plays tennis (figure 2.6). He plays effectively enough to go out and have fun at the local tennis club a couple of times per week and eventually decides to join a tennis league. Initially, it is just for fun, so he goes out and plays. Then he might decide to become competitive. Now it is not good enough to play effectively; he must also learn how to play more efficiently. The nervous system needs to learn how to coordinate movements better so that he can move faster on the court while still hitting the ball well and placing it out of reach of his opponent. The nervous system has to figure out how to do

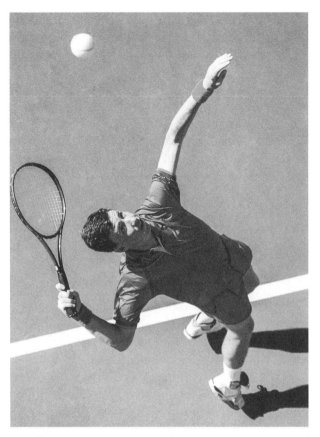

Figure 2.6 As his skill increases, a tennis player progresses from being effective to being efficient.

this consistently. He may be able to do this effectively if he can win a match, but not efficiently enough if he is so sore the next day he cannot win another match. Then to increase the efficiency, his nervous system needs to figure out how to either increase the resources available (get stronger, more flexible, faster) or to improve how it uses the resources (where to stand on the court, how to read the opponent better, be better coordinated, improve motor patterns).

There comes a point where we believe a given movement is efficient enough. When we can effectively accomplish the task at hand in an efficient manner, learning grinds to a halt. We then automatically repeat what we consider to be efficient, even though it could become more efficient if we continued to learn. This could be like the baby deciding to crawl through life. If we had to become more efficient we could, like the tennis player upping her game, but the cost–benefit ratio is too high. That is, it often requires too much time and effort for the nervous system, so learning essentially ends. The movement is effective and efficient enough, so we practice the task repetitively until it becomes habitual. Later in this book we examine how we get stuck in movement patterns that no longer serve us and how these habits can lead to injuries. For now, let's look at how to improve our movement abilities.

We are typically able to perform a task better through the combination of increasing available resources and improving how the resources are being used. When we face movement challenges, if it is important enough—if the cost–benefit ratio makes learning or improving a new skill worth it—we will figure out a way to do it. Both the baby learning to walk and the tennis player are being challenged. They become stronger, more balanced, and develop better muscle coordination over time. This holds true for everyday activities such as walking up and down stairs, squatting to plant a garden, and driving. If the challenge is not important enough to us, there is no reason for the nervous system to become more efficient or learn new activities.

We need to challenge our nervous system with meaningful movements if we want to stay active as we age. For us to learn something new or to improve on an activity in which we are already effective, we must give the nervous system puzzles. Solving problems makes us more efficient. From understanding this distinction between efficiency and effectiveness, we will move on to a third factor of movement: quality.

Quality of Movement

We have covered effective movement and efficient movement, but we need to define one more movement-related term: quality of movement. Quality of movement is an obscure expression—one of those "you know it when you see it" terms. We could say that certain athletes, dancers, and performers have it, but that does not help the adult who just wants to stay active. To say that you should move like Roger Federer on the tennis court or Fred Astaire on the dance floor is not a lot of help. By describing aspects of movement quality, we may be able to clarify what characteristics define quality of movement.

Different authors cite different aspects; for this book we use the following four characteristics to describe quality of movement:

1. It blends stability and mobility.
2. It is distributed throughout the body.
3. It is coordinated.
4. It is grounded.

Quality Movement Blends Stability and Mobility

Any movement combines stability and mobility. Stability is not usually absolute. It may mean an area of the body will be held still or move through a controlled pattern during a certain part of an action. When we blend stability and mobility, we are able to control the movement of different body parts, simultaneously holding still and allowing movement where appropriate.

A good example of blending steadiness and movement is the stable platform the shoulder blade provides when moving the arm. Without the stability of the shoulder blades, the upper extremities are at risk of injury during movement. This need for a stable platform has sometimes been misinterpreted as need for the shoulder blades to be held statically. This is not true. You should be able to control the shoulder blades when you are doing activities that involve the upper extremities without holding them rigidly in one position. For example, during yoga class it is often said that the shoulder blades should be held down and in. That is fine for early movements of the upper extremities, but once the arm is a bit below shoulder height, the shoulder needs to move and rotate. Otherwise the bone of the upper arm (humerus) and the tip of the shoulder (acromion) will bump into each other, pinching tendons that run between the shoulder blade and arm.

It is easy to see where an instruction like this has come from. Many people habitually use their upper trapezius when they raise their arms, which causes the shoulders to lift toward the ears. This elevates the shoulder blades and locks them in a position that prevents rotation as the arms are lifted, possibly leading to a shoulder impingement. So keeping the shoulder blades down and in is a well-meant instruction and appropriate for the early stages of the movement, but not for the later aspect of raising the arms overhead. The following movement exploration demonstrates the distinction in quality of movement.

EXPLORATION
Stability and Mobility

1 Try to lift your arms out to the sides and up overhead while at the same time using the upper trapezius to lift your shoulders toward your ears. Comfortable? Not likely.

2 Repeat, but this time with the shoulder blades held down and in. That is not very comfortable either because neither of these variations allow the shoulder blades to participate in the rhythm of the movement.

3 Now stabilize your shoulder blades down and in, lift your arms straight out to about 60 degrees, then allow your shoulder blades to participate in the movement as you continue to lift your arms overhead. Can you feel how you started lifting your arms from a stable platform (shoulder blades) and then allowed movement to occur in the shoulder blades? This is a good example of the blend of stability and mobility that is a characteristic of good movement: controlling the movement of different body parts, stabilizing, and allowing movement to occur as needed.

Quality Movement Is Distributed Throughout the Body

Every efficient movement should involve the whole body. Some parts of the body will occasionally be stable to allow efficient movements to occur, but eventually all body parts will be involved in an efficient movement. A movement that is isolated to one joint or one small part of the body is not efficient or strong and could eventually lead to arthritis in the joint that is overused. Even as I (Staffan) am typing this, there is movement throughout my body. As I reach my fingers toward certain keys, my body will rotate a bit. The reach is coming from my sitting bones if I am sitting or my feet if I am standing. Try it for yourself in the following movement exploration.

EXPLORATION
Typing

1 Type using only your fingers or forearms. Keep the rest of the body stiff. How long can you keep this up?

2 Continue this as you hold your breath. Is it comfortable?

3 Breathe and allow the rest of your body to participate in the typing. Notice the difference. How does the breath move the spine and involve it in the typing action? How often do you hold your breath, or breathe very shallowly, when you are typing or doing something else that requires concentration? Paying attention to the breath automatically softens your body and allows more of the body to participate. Paying attention to the breath also ties into the previous principle of allowing a combination of mobility and stability. When you inhale, the body becomes more stable and when you exhale you allow more mobility. That is why in yoga, twists tend to be performed on the out-breath. The body allows for more mobility on the out-breath.

Quality Movement Is Coordinated

Good movement quality shows coordination. In movement, muscles are categorized as agonists, antagonists, and stabilizers. The agonist muscle shortens and moves the joint, the antagonist muscle relaxes and lengthens to allow the movement, and the stabilizer muscle creates a secure platform on which movement can happen efficiently. Think about what happens when you bend your elbow. The biceps muscle is the agonist and flexes the joint, the triceps is the antagonist and relaxes so it doesn't fight the movement of the biceps and elbow, and the muscles around the shoulder blade stabilize. If the triceps muscle does not relax and lengthen when the elbow flexes, the movement is not well coordinated. The body is working against itself. This is a simplified and isolated way to look at coordination. Much more is going on in a well-coordinated movement as the muscles are engaged throughout the body, but for our purposes it is enough to think about the main muscles involved in movement and stability.

Quality Movement Is Grounded

A good quality of movement is grounded. You may wonder how grounded the dancer who floats above the ground is, but what is meant here is the person is aware of the ground and knows how to use it. A dancer or athlete pushes off the ground in order to perform amazing feats in the air. They are also aware of the ground before they land, are grounded in their own bodies, and know how the ground and the body perform together. They use the ground for efficient, graceful movements. The following exercise lets you explore your relationship to the ground.

This is grounding. Know how you and the ground interact. Sense the grounding in your body. This is important when you start doing the asanas later in this book as well as in any activity you perform. Have you ever thought about how you use the ground when you are walking? Play with it!

A quality movement blends stability and mobility, is distributed through the body, is coordinated, and is grounded. Effective, efficient, quality movements set the stage for a long, healthy, active life.

EXPLORATION

Grounded-Movement

1 Sit in a chair. Come to standing. What happened under your feet when you stood up?

2 Do it again, this time paying attention to what happens in your feet when you stand up.

3 Sit down again, and then stand up while pushing the feet into the ground. Do you notice the difference?

4 Repeat one more time, but now lift your toes off the ground as you come to standing. How was this variation different?

Learning New Activities and Improving Old Ones

When the nervous system solves the puzzle of a new activity, we go through certain predictable steps. Learning can be divided into three stages:

1. Cognitive
2. Associative
3. Autonomous

In the cognitive stage, your movements are slow and inefficient, even though they might still be effective. You move stiffly because you are decreasing the degrees of freedom. That is to say, the nervous system is trying to stiffen as many joints as possible so that it doesn't have to coordinate the actions of many different muscles.

Think about a person learning how to ice skate. The new skater tightens as many muscles as possible and looks stiff, tight, and clumsy because she really has to think about how to do the movement. Because there are few degrees of freedom, there is little variability in movement at the initial cognitive stage of learning. This learning phase is mentally and physically fatiguing.

As you move into the associative stage, there are more degrees of freedom available, so more of the body is involved in the movement. The movement is smoother and becomes more efficient because it does not take as much thinking or physical effort to perform. The person learning to skate may start to appear graceful and be better able to maneuver across the ice. The movement is not quite automatic though; that happens in stage three of learning.

The third stage, the autonomous, or motor stage, demonstrates precise movements. You reach the desired outcome in a consistent and efficient manner. You move smoothly and comfortably so there are more degrees of freedom, which means you can vary the movement more. The ice skater applies those available degrees of freedom to do pirouettes, jumps, and intricate footwork (figure 2.7) To perform

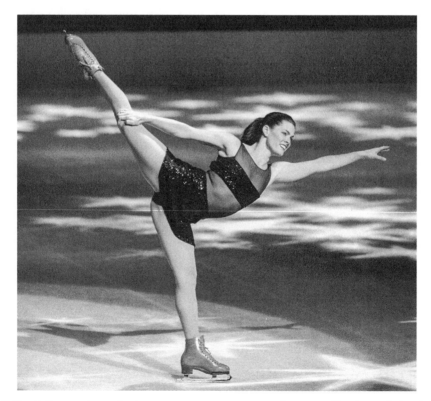

Figure 2.7 A figure skater in the autonomous stage performs well using minimal thought and effort.

advanced movements, you need to allow as many parts of the body as possible to participate in each action. This offers a lot of degrees of freedom! But what do you do after you have reached and mastered the autonomous stage of a movement?

At the autonomous stage, most people stop developing their movement skills. The movement is good enough and effective enough to accomplish the desired outcome consistently, so it becomes habitual and automatic. Why not continue to explore movements to make the desired actions even more efficient? To relearn a movement in a more efficient way requires you to go through all of the stages of learning again. Although sometimes the movement pattern needs a complete overhaul, typically each of the stages will not last as long as they initially did because all that is needed is a refinement of the basic movement pattern that has already been developed.

It is helpful to consider certain movement characteristics when you learn new movements and when you perform the yoga poses later in this book. To learn new movements or relearn old ones, try the following:

- Play with their reversibility.
- Slow them down.
- Experiment with balance.
- Make the movements independent from your head and neck.
- Involve your breath.
- Focus on the lengthening (antagonist) muscle.
- Remain fully aware.

Reversibility

When you are practicing a new movement or want to improve a habitual pattern, try to practice the movement in a controlled, reversible way. That is, you should be able to stop the movement at any time and reverse it.

In the Western world, walking is described as controlled falling. In the martial arts world, on the other hand, walking is about not falling. The martial artist is in control of movements at all times. The body weight is within the base of support, and weight will not transfer to the stepping foot until it is safely touching the ground. Compare that technique to the style of walking where body weight moves forward outside the base of support before the stepping foot is on the ground, leading to the body falling forward onto the stepping foot.

Now get up and try these two ways of walking. Can you stop midstep and reverse your stride? Rather than automatically pacing through controlled falling, you have to be keenly aware of the dynamics of stability, mobility, and balance throughout the body when you walk in a controlled, reversible way.

Body Organization

We use the term body organization throughout this book as a way to describe the position of the whole body and the relationship between parts of the body. To move in an efficient way the body must be organized so that it can perform the task at hand without any unnecessary strain, or be ready to move in any direction without any unnecessary extra preparation.

This short exploration gives you an idea of how to organize the body to move towards a position where you can move with equal ease. Body organization is

EXPLORATION

Body Organization in Mountain Pose

1 Stand with the feet parallel and hip width apart. Distribute the weight equally between the outer and inner edge of the foot, and the front and back of the foot.

2 Let your arms hang by your sides, with the palms facing forward if possible. If it causes too much strain to fully turn your palms forward, then turn them forward as much as possible without straining.

3 Align your head with your spine. Slightly pull the chin in towards the neck. Move your shoulder blades slightly down and in towards the thoracic spine.

4 Notice which muscles in your legs are more engaged. Are they the quadriceps muscles in the front of the thighs, or the hamstrings in the back of your thighs?

5 Without adjusting your stance, predict if it would be easier to take a step forward or backwards? Would it be easier to move to the left or right? To pivot to the left or right?

6 Now gently rock back and forth on your feet. Can you feel that as you put more weight on the front of your feet you are more ready to move forward, and the muscles in the back of your leg tighten? As you put more weight on the back part of your feet, do the muscles in the front of the leg tighten up and do you feel more ready to take a step back?

7 Now find your sweet spot. That is where you have equal muscle tension in the front and backs of your legs, and there is equal pressure from your whole foot on the ground.

8 Can you sense that in this position you are ready to take a step forward or back with equal ease?

9 Now play with swaying from side to side until you are equally ready to take a step to the left as you are to step to the right.

10 Then combine the side-to-side swaying with the forward-back movement, until you can step forward, backward, or to either side with equal ease and without having to adjust your body before stepping in either direction.

different from posture in that in good posture we cannot move in either direction with equal ease. Throughout the book we will bring up the idea of optimal body organization again and again. We will also talk about body organization when we talk about emotions, since each emotion has a different body organization. Think about the slouched posture of a depressed person, or the upright posture of someone who is proud and uplifted. In yoga, good examples of this are how we organize our body in warrior 1 and warrior 2 (chapter 10). We have a strong stance; we organize ourselves so that we are grounded and strong. Arms are up, head is aligned with the spine, and the gaze is focused. We have organized our bodies so that we feel strong. Compare this to child's pose, where we are curled up, belly towards the ground. We feel safe and nurtured in that body organization. Body organization is more than posture. It is the pattern of the whole body that allows us to move efficiently in any direction, but we can also use body organization to evoke certain emotions.

Slow Movement

When you learn a new movement it is important to perform it slowly so that the nervous system can fully sense the action. Sensors called proprioceptors tell us where we are in space. Proprioceptors provide information to the CNS about muscle length, tension, and joint angle. The CNS uses this information about where the body is in space to determine which muscles to use for stability or mobility, which ones to lengthen, and which ones to shorten. With repetition, this stored information can be readily used in the future to avoid injuries when the body is organized in the same way and in the same context. The CNS has learned what to do and can send the same orders quickly. Conversely, if the movement is performed quickly during the learning phase, the CNS will not register it in the same way and might not be able to react as quickly the next time the body is organized in the same way. Even movements that are performed quickly need the initial slow practice. In martial arts such as tai chi, movements are performed slowly but can eventually be used at full speed in combat. Once the timing and procedure of the movement have been mastered in a slow fashion, you can pick up the pace and eventually do it at full speed.

Balance

In this context, balance is closely related to controlled reversibility and slow movement. Without balance, reversibility and slow movement are impossible to perform. Many times people cannot move in a slow or reversible way because of poor balance. So what is balance?

Most people think of balance as being able to maintain a posture in a steady manner, but balance can mean many things. When we are learning a movement, we do not produce it perfectly right away. In the cognitive and associative stages we likely lose stability, fail to perform the movement in an aesthetically pleasing way, or are ineffective in our judgement and decision of how to produce the action. Despite this, can you still maintain balance? That is, can you maintain mental and emotional stability when you lose your physical balance? Can you decide to try again? If you can, then you are maintaining balance.

If you believe that you will lose your balance every time you can't maintain a posture, it is easy to get discouraged and stop trying to learn new movements. In the *Yoga Sutras*, yoga is defined as quieting the waves of the mind, maintaining mental and emotional stability. That internal stability is related to balancing the body. As a movement characteristic, let us maintain this wider definition of balance.

Freedom of the Head

People don't often think about freedom of the head as a movement characteristic. During the first stage of learning, you decrease the degrees of freedom in the body to create a sense of stability. Proprioceptors are sensing from inside your ears, and by stabilizing the head and neck and fixing your eyes on the horizon, you gain a sense of steadiness. As you become more competent, you can differentiate the movement of the head and neck from the rest of the body. Look at high-level athletes: They can stabilize the head on top of a moving body, or turn the head and eyes to locate other players while still performing the physical skills of the game. For anyone who wants to stay active, it is important to differentiate the head and neck from the body. This differentiation is important in athletic activities, driving, housework, or finding out who called your name in a crowded mall without falling down when turning your head.

Breathing

Holding your breath impairs movement. Yoga emphasizes the breath. Flexion, or bending a joint, tends to be coupled with the out-breath, and extension, opening a joint, tends to be coupled with the in-breath. Holding your breath when you learn a movement indicates either habitual breath-holding or the nervous system trying to decrease the degrees of freedom. In competitive weight lifting, this stability may be beneficial. However, in most cases you tend to be more skillful if you can maintain smooth, free breathing.

Length

Movements should create length in the body, especially in the spine. Both Pilates and yoga emphasize length. This might seem counterintuitive because people tend to focus on the muscle that shortens when they perform a movement, but when there is a shortening muscle (agonist) there is also a lengthening muscle (antagonist). If you focus on the lengthening muscle, your perception of the movement tends to change and you get a sense of length in the body. While it is valuable to focus on the agonist, much can be gained by being aware of length and the antagonist action.

Awareness

Reversibility, slow movement, balance, freedom from the head, breathing, and length all require awareness of how you are moving. Any well-performed movement requires focused attention while you learn or improve it. The concept of awareness is central to yoga therapy, and we come back to its importance repeatedly in this book.

Unless you are a high-level athlete, dancer, manual laborer, or someone else who uses the body to make a living, you will not spend hours every day refining your movements. You might not be able to perform a certain action because of injury, illness, aging, or just plain inactivity. You will have to relearn movements, and if you have not performed movement explorations since you were young, it will be difficult to learn new or varied movements. Wouldn't it be better if you explored new and exciting movement possibilities throughout your life instead of waiting until you are forced to do it? Imagine waking up every morning or taking short breaks at work and challenging your brain to explore new movement patterns. By practicing yoga therapy, we give you the chance to move through the three stages of learning and apply the seven features of movement refinement.

Importance of Exploring Movement

Now we know why it is important to move efficiently and to learn new movements or modify patterned ones. Although it is time consuming, it is important to explore movements throughout life, not just as children learning to walk, ride a bike, or catch a ball. There are several good reasons why we should invest time and effort in continued exploration of movement.

It's Fun

It feels good to learn something new. The main way babies learn is through their body, through physical experiences such as grasping, crawling, sitting, standing, walking, speaking, and so on. To an adult it can be frustrating to learn a new skill, but look at the joyous surprise babies experience the first time they figure out how to stand, before they fall down again, that is! Children whose nervous system solves the puzzle of balance on a bicycle are also exalted. Even though there is something important and exhilarating about learning through the body, as adults we remove ourselves further and further from that excitement. Instead, we limit ourselves by avoiding many actions and places where we would be forced to learn a new activity. We might even limit our beliefs, feeling like we are too old to learn something new. Maybe we should change the old adage to "You can teach an old dog new tricks, and how to enjoy learning them."

When it comes to adult learning, we now know that with the correct input and environment, the brain will keep learning, making new neuronal connections, and changing the size and shape of the brain (neuroplasticity). Just 20 years ago we had a limited view of when the brain stops developing. Recent research into neuroplasticity indicates that the nervous system can learn to rewire much later in life than we thought possible, especially if there is a sense of fun around it.

To change the brain and nervous system, you need to learn through your body, as you did when you were young. You need to feel the joy of learning a new skill, no matter what your age. The nervous system thrives on learning; there is nothing healthier for it than to learn a new activity or way to perform it. We believe that one of the reasons so many people enjoy yoga is that they learn something new with their bodies. A new asana, something they didn't think they could do. You can see the joy and pride when people leave the yoga studio after they have accomplished something previously beyond their limits, something they may have thought was outside of their abilities. The fun of learning something new is a key reason to put in the effort.

It's Healthy to Challenge the Movement System

All three components of the movement system benefit from challenge. We know it is healthy for the nervous system to learn something new, but it is also great for the muscles and skeleton. The muscles get stronger and more flexible, which offsets the stiffness and weakness that comes from aging and inactivity. Yoga will work those muscles, and the flexibility and strength will come back. Yoga and movement are also good for the skeletal system. The bones become stronger when we put weight on them. With osteoporosis a concern in the Western world, strengthening the bones through yoga and movement is something that we should all do. The nervous system, the muscles, and the skeleton all need to be challenged through movement so that we can continue to grow and stay active.

It Decreases the Chance of Overuse Injuries

More and more adults are staying active into their later years. Whether that is through walking, hiking, playing golf, running, or any other activity that brings them joy, people want to stay active. Many of these activities, however, involve repetitive movements. If a person gets injured and only has one habitual way of doing repetitive movements, then he will keep bumping into the pain over and over again. The movement system does not have an alternative solution to the movement problem. If, on the other hand, the person has played with and explored a variety of movements, the movement system has the flexibility to solve the problem. It can adjust the movement so that the pain is avoided or minimized. In later chapters we discuss how to prevent injuries and use movement variations to prevent repeated injuries.

Exploring movement patterns is important in staying active through the life span because it's fun and healthy and decreases the risk of overuse injuries. Yoga therapy offers the chance to experience this kind of play. Yoga further helps you improve the efficiency of activities beyond your yoga practice.

Improving the Efficiency of Activities

It might seem counterintuitive that yoga can improve your ability to perform many seemingly unrelated activities. Improved strength and flexibility are a couple of reasons why this is so. But, perhaps more important, yoga gives the nervous system puzzles to solve. Yoga asanas force you to organize the body in ways you are not used to. How do you find a posture you have never been in before? How do you maintain balance when the proprioceptors are not lined up? How do you keep breathing deeply when challenged? How do you maintain a calm mind while you struggle? (After all, yoga therapy requires a stable mind and stable body.) Once the movement system has solved the problems in yoga poses, you can see the effect. After practice, do an activity that you enjoy; you may find new options for movement. Try an activity that you have difficulty with and you will be amazed that it feels easier. Why is this?

There may be many reasons why an activity suddenly feels easier or more efficient after asana practice. Our belief comes back to the movement system, especially the nervous system, learning something new when performing asanas. Once the movement and nervous systems have learned, they incorporate aspects of that new movement into other activities. This is amplified if you perform the activities soon after the yoga practice.

One of the beautiful aspects of yoga therapy is that it challenges the nervous system to organize the body outside of the habitual manner. Yoga therapy combines this new organization with awareness and increased mind–body sensitivity to create powerful opportunities to learn, build effectiveness, and enjoy life more. Yoga therapy incorporates all the key points of efficient learning, with special prowess in slow movements and focusing on the breath.

You can only transfer new movement skills to old activities if you are aware of the movement while learning it and incorporate it in new activities as soon as possible. When you are aware, you feel that the movement or activity is different after you do the asana practice than it was before. Without awareness, you move in the habitual way. Slowing down gives you a chance to reflect and become aware.

Slow movements are more meditative and introspective, offering time to observe passing thoughts, how you move or rest, and how thoughts and movements relate. Today, too many people are stressed and overly influenced by the SNS. For healing and learning to take place, you need to dampen its effect and allow the PNS to have more influence. Slowing the breath and coordinating it with movement helps this happen. While vigorous asanas paired with breath can have this effect, slow movements and slow coordinated breathing are more efficient in healing and learning new movement. If you choose a vigorous practice, remain aware of why you are performing it. If it is for a workout, that's great. If you wish to learn and challenge your nervous system, a slower, mindful practice will bring more benefit. Maybe slowing down will give you a chance to observe how stressed you are and how good you can feel when you perform asanas and slow movements with coordinated breathing and awareness.

No matter what form of yoga you practice, do not cut the corpse pose (savasana) short (figure 2.8). Frequently people hurry off the mat without taking 5 to 10 minutes to complete the ultimate phase of a yoga session, that wonderful corpse pose. It might be the only time all day that you can actually let go of everything and allow the nervous system to rest. The silence lets our PNS take over for the SNS and allows healing and learning to take place. In relaxation, the nervous system incorporates some of the new body organizations and movement sequences that you just performed. Savasana also gives you time for self-reflection—something that is important in yoga therapy. In addition, you leave the session with a sense of peace and calm. How long can you maintain that peace and calm of the dominant PNS? Simply by noticing this different state of mind and body, you will become more aware of when the SNS is activating and then guide yourself back to relaxation. This will improve your efficiency, quality of movement, and learning.

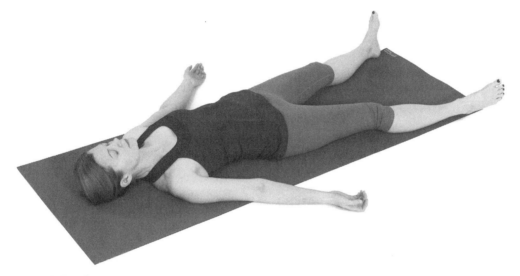

Figure 2.8   Corpse pose.

It is our hope that by now you have an idea about our approach to yoga therapy. We look at it as a form of learning for the whole movement system: muscles, bones, and nervous system. Our focus tends to be on the nervous system. We believe it is best to practice a variety of asanas and movement sequences, and that actions should be performed with coordination between the movement, breath, and awareness. We further believe that by paying attention to how you practice yoga and knowing the characteristics of efficient movement and conditions for learning, you are ready to explore how you can stay active for the rest of your life. Staying active means enjoying the activities you want to and keeping the nervous system happy and ready to respond. That is how to live life to its fullest. We hope you use yoga therapy as a way to explore and reflect on how you can stay active with greater ease and efficiency. We will address much more about yoga therapy practices, and how you can vary them so that there is always a new challenge for your nervous system. The next steps are to identify, differentiate, and integrate!

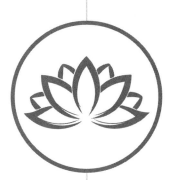

three
Connecting Brain to Body

If life had to be summarized in just one concept, it would be movement. To live is to keep moving. It is a cycle of activity and rest, and even when we are at rest, movement takes place inside of and all around us.

Have you ever thought about all of the movements that you perform in one day? Are they varied? How many times do you think you repeat the same movement pattern in one day? A week? A month? A year? How many of those movements are done with awareness? Do you choose how you will perform them, or do you just do them? What is the difference between choosing and not choosing, and why should you even care? A principle in the field of somatic (relating to bodily sensations and perceptions) education, which we will explore in this chapter, offers compelling food for thought on this subject:

Undifferentiated Movement = Undifferentiated Perception = Undifferentiated Thinking

That's bad news if you've never thought about differentiating your movement patterns. The good news is that the opposite is also true:

Differentiated Movement = Differentiated Perception = Differentiated Thinking

And you are already on your way to differentiating your movement patterns by engaging with this book. Cultivating varied movement practices will improve the daily experience of your active life and increase your ability to continue to move and live as you age.

This chapter introduces the field of somatic education and how it can influence what you do during asana practice, leading to safer and more pleasurable activities on and off the yoga mat. We introduce the concepts of **identification, differentiation,** and **integration** as the foundations for therapeutic yoga movement practices. As an active adult who wants to develop more efficient movements and skills, you must first identify habitual movement patterns. Once identified, develop the ability to differentiate those movements into various options. Differentiation itself is not enough, though; in the end, you integrate the nonhabitual movement options into your repertoire. This chapter also discusses how habitual movement patterns can limit progress, decrease efficacy of chosen activities, and lead to injury.

Yoga Therapy and Somatic Education

Have you heard the proverb about a group of blind men encountering an elephant for the first time and trying to figure out what it is? One man touches the leg and says, "It is thick and heavy, it must be a tree trunk." Another man grasps the ear and says, "It is thin, but strong and flexible. It must be a leaf." Another finds the tail and argues, "No, it is a rope," while another touches the trunk and says, "You are all wrong; it is a large snake." The man on the side of the elephant says, "I don't know what you all are talking about. I am touching the side of a mountain." These blind men are all correct, but continue to argue with each another because of the difference in their points of view. Similarly, the field of yoga therapy has many perspectives and, subsequently, different approaches toward healing based on those perspectives.

The various definitions of yoga therapy are often based on a combination of many factors: ethnic and cultural background; previous training in other fields, such as psychology, medicine, physiology, and philosophy; the perspective of our teachers; and our personal experience of yoga. Influences from media, friends, family, society, and other sources also play roles.

The person with a background in yoga might define *yoga* therapy from the point of view of her favorite style of yoga that has been adapted to solicit therapeutic benefits. The person who is less experienced with yoga might approach yoga *therapy* based on her previous experience with the subject–object model discussed in chapter 1, in which the doctor or therapist is paid to "fix" the patient.

It is important to us that you consider what yoga therapy means to you. Is it a spiritual quest? Is it a lifestyle? Is it education? Does it improve your strength? Your mobility? Your sensitivity to self? Let yourself hang out with the question of what yoga therapy means to you while you are engaging with and integrating the materials that we offer. Your definition can and should evolve with your needs and experiences.

Everyone comes to yoga with ideas about what it is or at least what they want yoga therapy to help them with. It could be pain or an injury that motivates them, a need for socialization or connectedness, a way to sort out difficult emotions, or a quest for meaning and purpose in their lives. They have seen or heard about a part of the elephant that is yoga therapy and want what that part of the elephant can bring them. At this point they have a choice to either get caught up in arguing about "what the elephant is" or simply agree that the elephant has many parts, and that each aspect of the elephant is valid and worth exploring. Yoga is vast, and that vastness lends itself to different people finding different meanings and being served by different aspects of the elephant.

Our perspective is that it is important to look at yoga therapy as a means of challenging the movement system with puzzles. Learning to solve movement problems makes you more sensitive and aware of yourself, which in turn leads to changes in how you accomplish things, relate to others, and reflect inward. It may even lead to a spiritual understanding of how your life unfolds. It is our hope that as you start to touch different parts of the yoga therapy elephant by challenging your movement system, you will stay open to examining other aspects as well. However, the main focus of this book is the movement system. Remember, the movement system interacts with every other system in your body, so be ready for surprises. Yoga therapy reaches into many areas of life, even when you focus on only one specific realm.

The term yoga therapy might be misleading. In this book we suggest that although it is therapeutic, it is an educational process. In school, learning tends to follow a certain pattern: The teacher lectures on a topic and then presents the student with a problem to solve. You can look at yoga therapy in the same way. If you see it as a way to solve puzzles and improve awareness of your actions and internal senses, yoga therapy fits into an educational model. Because yoga includes physical, mental, and emotional processes, it fits the model of somatic education.

Somatic education includes practices such as biofeedback, relaxation techniques, the Feldenkrais method, the Alexander technique, Rolfing, Laban, nia, tai chi, and eutony. Somatics is a term first used by Thomas Hanna in 1986 in a three-part series of articles he wrote for the journal *Somatics*. Hanna defined somatics as "the art and science of the inter-relational process between awareness, biological functioning, and the environment, all three factors being identified as a synergistic whole." Hanna chose the word soma instead of body because he felt that body was something fixed, or static, in most people's minds. Soma, according to Hanna, stands for the living, ever-changing body.

Hanna's definition of somatics may sound familiar to yoga practitioners. In yoga, we talk about the koshas (layers of a being), and how the koshas interact with each other. Koshas philosophy states that all humans are made up of five layers: the physical body; breath and life energy; senses, feelings, and thoughts; intellect; and spirit. The interactions and integration of the koshas lead to a synergistic whole—the same synergistic whole that is central to somatics and is present when we are doing an activity well. Hannah's definition is not the only one in the field of somatics that echoes the field of yoga therapy.

Another somatic educator and Feldenkrais practitioner, Yvan Joly, defines the soma as the sum of the body's subjective lived experiences, including thoughts, emotions, and fantasies, the totality of our biological and neurological processes (Joly 2001). The emphasis here is on the lived experience. Joly does not perceive the body as an object that is probed and examined. His theory should sound familiar to yoga therapists who understand movement and awareness as key concepts in yoga practice. According to Joly, somatic education has four central aspects:

1. **Movement.** Movement equals life. All schools of yoga agree with that statement to some extent. You move. You are alive. Even if you are sitting in meditation, your breath and organs move.

2. **Awareness of the living body from the inside.** You self-regulate and organize based on the input you get from your body. In yoga, you do this as you move in and out of asanas, becoming more sensitive to the input you are getting from your internal senses. You might start a meditation practice to meet some of your needs based on this self-regulating awareness. While early on in your yoga practice you might be guided by a teacher, there often comes a point where you become so aware of your internal sensations that you practice based on your sensations, rhythms, and internal needs. At that point, your self-awareness does not come from a teacher, mirror, or other external point; awareness comes from inside your own body.

3. **Learning.** You know that learning has occurred when you see a change in actions and behavior. While some learning may take place at an intellectual level, for somatic learning to occur there must be an observable change in behavior. When you learn somatically, the way you perform your daily activities changes; they are easier and more enjoyable. You are more likely to take on difficult new activities or are determined to become proficient at an activity. You develop tapas (discipline) because you enjoy learning and taking on challenges.

4. **Space.** Your somatic experience is influenced by the space around it. In other words, you embody your soma through the environment. You may find that after reading this book and developing your own movement practice, you act differently. You are kinder to yourself and others, adopt new routines at work and at home, or eat and sleep better. These embodied environmental changes allow you to be more focused, active, and efficient doing the things that you enjoy. Sustained yoga practice doesn't initiate change in just one area of your life. Just like you can't work on one kosha without influencing all the others, change in one area of life affects all other areas. With carefully guided, mindful yoga practice, you change toward health and balance in all areas of your life. As yoga author and educator Leslie Kaminoff wrote in one of his blog posts, "Yoga is inherent movement toward equilibrium." We change toward balance in all aspects of life. Once we have found equilibrium through balanced practice, all of our activities become much more enjoyable.

The definitions of somatic education and yoga therapy are similar. Somatic education does not differentiate between physical, psychological, and emotional states. The somatic education practitioner looks at the totality of the student, just like the yoga therapist does. The yoga therapist might look at the five koshas, while the somatic educator looks at the combined sum of the physical, psychological, and emotional states; however, the underlying holistic philosophy is the same. It might sound strange to claim that there is no difference between physical, psychological, and emotional states, and many professionals would argue against this idea. After all, if this were the case, we would not need psychologists, physical therapists, or occupational therapists, but is this claim about a synergistic whole really so outrageous?

Every day we use body language as a cue to people's mental and emotional states. Body language is a known aspect of communication. When we speak body language, we are often able to decode a situation or understand a person better than if we were using spoken language. Simply by observing a person's stance, how a person moves his extremities or orients himself in the environment, we learn about how he perceives a situation. This allows us to respond more effectively and compassionately. A big clue into people's moods is their movements and posture. Although you may not have realized it at the time, you have probably been aware of a person's whole, synergistic self when, before even talking to her, you could tell whether she was happy or depressed. How did you differentiate that? How quickly or slowly did she cross a room? What was her spinal posture? How big were her gestures? We read the physical, psychological, and emotional states of people all the time, often without conscious analysis. We just do it. The more cognizant we are of body language, the more we are connected to a person's whole being.

The body language exercise gives you the opportunity to differentiate your own emotional states through the expression of your body. Have fun playing with this exercise and experimenting with the results in everyday life.

A key premise of somatic education is that each emotional state has a corresponding body organization. The somatic educator can guide the student in recognizing how the body organizes itself based on emotional occurrences and then offer new options. When you move in nonhabitual ways and organize the body around certain emotions, the nervous system has more choices for solving emotional puzzles, and you do not have to respond to emotional situations in a habitual way.

Another problem for the nervous system to solve is how to improve performance in certain activities, such as specific sports or recovering from injury. The somatic

EXPLORATION

Body Language

1 In a standing position, raise your arms overhead as if you had just won an Olympic gold medal. What happens to your face? Do your eyes open wider? Maybe you notice a smile? How do you feel? Happy? Confident? Like a winner?

2 Do the same thing, but before you raise your arms, frown and make a sad face. How does that feel? Do you feel like a winner? Did your mood change? Is it more difficult to lift your arms?

3 Sit down and slouch. Let your head hang in your best imitation of a depressed person. What happens to your face? Does your forehead wrinkle? Do you feel like a winner?

4 Now come back to a seated posture. Smile a big, genuine smile. Open your eyes wide. Then slouch into your depressed posture without changing your face. Do you feel depressed? Is it more difficult to slouch with a smile on your face? Isn't it interesting how much our body affects our mood and vice versa?

educator facilitates this by guiding people toward a body organization that is unfamiliar to the nervous system, thereby giving the nervous system more options for how to improve the desired performance. When the nervous system, muscles, and bones have many options for solving a movement puzzle, it improves your ability to perform the (possibly unrelated) desired activity.

This somatic education process is not far from yoga therapy. Yoga therapists suggest asanas that organize the body in a manner that is unfamiliar to the nervous system. In addition to presenting the nervous system with the physical puzzle, the asana might also present an emotional challenge. For one who lacks confidence, it might be a yoga posture that also involves raising the chest and arms into the air, such as a tree pose. For someone who is overly busy, perhaps it is a challenge to do a child's pose, resting the forehead on the floor. Yoga therapy serves as a somatic education tool.

A skillful yoga therapist or somatic educator will take you through the various stages of a movement and explain how you can add variations to allow for different experiences. No matter what asana or activity you do, be aware that you are always working on, and with, the synchronous whole. Although it's tempting to separate parts from the whole, the idea of separation is an illusion, albeit a comforting one. People have been taught to see the body as a machine with separate parts that function together, rather than as a functioning interactive whole. This mechanistic view of the body may be helpful in some circumstances; however, when you seek longevity through the movement system, you must instead consider integrated functioning, and take a holistic view.

A holistic view of the body helps you create more movement options. The foundation of your chosen activity forms around an increased awareness of how you can introduce variety to it. You can adapt the activity to what you need each day. If you listen to your present needs through your internal senses, the way you perform an asana today might not be exactly the way you did it yesterday or the way you will do it tomorrow. Some days you might need to perform the asana slower to enhance the emotional sensation, or create intricate variety to challenge your nervous system, or be more spiritual by keeping your extremities close to your torso. In chapter 8 we give examples of how you can vary the asanas so that they fit your current needs, and how they can work with the kosha that you want to put in the foreground of that day's practice. Please note that even though one kosha is in the foreground, the others are still involved in the background because you are exploring options with the awareness that you are a synchronized whole.

Skillful yoga therapists can also work with the synchronized whole of your being. They can move you through a range of emotions and neurological puzzles in a session or have you stay and explore a single emotion or neurological puzzle. It is the *organization* of the soma—the living, changing body—that evokes the sensations and emotions that create the puzzles for the movement system to solve. This holistic approach ultimately supports the longevity of healthy movement and a healthy nervous system through your lifespan. When the session is over, you then integrate what was learned into your life and daily activities.

EXPLORATION
Asana Movement

❶ For safety, stand behind a chair or kitchen counter in case you lose your balance. Lift your right foot off the floor and put the sole on the side of your left calf to balance on the left foot.

❷ On the in-breath, raise your arms overhead. What do you feel? Can you allow the sensations to rise in you as you stand there while also using the nervous system to solve the balance puzzle and sense the contact of the right foot against the left leg? Can you sense the emotion while you are challenged to keep your balance?

❸ You can make the puzzle more challenging for the movement system by closing your eyes. Now the nervous system has to completely depend on internal feedback. When you closed your eyes and had to focus so hard on the movement challenge, did you lose your sense of the emotional aspect?

❹ Repeat the tree pose, but put your hands in the prayer position, with palms together in front of the chest. Now what do you experience? Is it a similar exhilarating feeling, or something more peaceful? Is it easier or more difficult to find your balance with the hands in prayer position?

Identification, Differentiation, and Integration

You can see that yoga and somatic education have much in common. Do you remember the principle of somatic education that we offered in the beginning of this chapter?

Undifferentiated Movement = Undifferentiated Perception = Undifferentiated Thinking

Differentiated Movement = Differentiated Perception = Differentiated Thinking

How do you differentiate these aspects of your being to improve your movements, perceptions, thinking, and life? The first step is identification.

Identification

The first thing you need to do when you want to improve a movement is to identify what you are already doing. Often when you go to the personal trainer, physical therapist, chiropractor, or yoga teacher, you are asked to move differently than your habitual pattern dictates. You may be instructed on how to change your movement to improve performance, decrease pain, or stabilize the body. You leave the clinic with an idea of how you should move based on feedback from the facilitator or the correct movement you saw in the mirror. However, you are rarely shown the original, habitual movement. Do you know the internal feeling of the habitual movement you are trying to correct or improve? Unless you can identify how you are performing the movement that you want to improve or change, how can you improve or change it?

If you don't know what you are doing, you can't do what you want.
—Moshe Feldenkrais

Larry Goldfarb, a pioneering practitioner of the Feldenkrais method, uses the Paris subway as a metaphor for what happens when someone tries to change a movement without first identifying it: When you emerge from the subway, there is usually a map that will help you figure out where you are going. It has a dot that says, "You are here." Based on where you are on the map, you can figure out how to get to where you want to go. Sometimes, someone has played a prank and removed the dot indicating where you are. Without knowing where you are, how can you get where you want to go? The map becomes useless. As such, your ability to make sustainable changes is reduced when you learn new movements or modify old habits without identifying how you are already performing the movement.

Unless you can recognize your present movement pattern, it is difficult to change it. To see how you move or perform an action by looking in a mirror is helpful, but not sufficient. You also need to be able to recognize the internal feeling that occurs during the movement. When you are aware of your body from this internal sense and able to use it in skilled ways, we call it kinesthetic intelligence.

Kinesthetic intelligence is an integral part of yoga therapy. The yoga therapist might ask you to exaggerate a movement habit you want to change so that you can sense it at a kinesthetic level. Even though it is counterintuitive to do more of what you don't want to do, exaggerating the movement to increase bodily awareness is like marking where you are on the map. Once you have identified the movement at a kinesthetic level, you will recognize it when you are active and can choose to move in a different way. You know where you are on the map and can now chart the course to where you want to go. That is, you can differentiate and create options in how you perform an activity.

The following movement exploration and associated questions for reflection will help you understand how to identify your movement patterns.

You can go through this identification process with any activities that you do habitually, especially those that you want to change and improve. The first step toward differentiation is always to identify what you are doing. Know where you are starting. The next step is differentiating the movement into various choices.

EXPLORATION

Identification

1 Start in a tabletop position on all fours with your knees directly under your hips and your hands directly under your shoulders. Now round your spine toward the ceiling (the cat movement). Allow your head to drop toward the floor as you do this (a).

2 On the next breath allow your belly to sink toward the floor and your head to rise up toward the ceiling as far as is comfortable (the cow movement) (b).

3 On the next breath repeat step 1. How did you perform the movement? Do you know where you started it? Was it the head? Lower back? Midback? Did you round your back on the in-breath or the out-breath, or did you hold your breath? Did you have more weight on your hands or your knees? On your right side or left side? All these variables are part of identification.

4 Go back and do this asana sequence again. Pay attention to what you are actually doing. Don't try to change anything. Just do it the way you usually do and notice what that is.

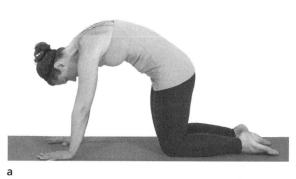

a

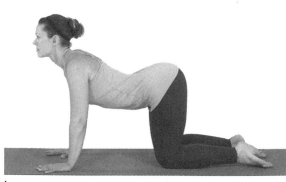

b

Differentiation

After you have identified your habitual movement patterns, it is time to differentiate them. If you want to grow, you have to change your patterns. This may mean taking small risks and moving outside your comfort zone. A lot of emotions arise when you change your patterns. Through differentiation, you can develop options for a specific movement, asana, or activity. The following exercise guides you through a differentiation process.

What do these differentiations do for you? By now you can probably guess the answer to that question. They create puzzles for the nervous system to solve. On a more practical level, through differentiation you become more responsive to your environment. When you have options, you can apply different movement choices depending on what happens around you and the information you get from your internal senses. You notice the difference between various patterns.

In the identification phase, you learn how it feels when you move in the habitual manner. In the differentiation phase, you learn how to create and recognize movement options. It is important to be able to feel differences at the kinesthetic level because movement is an internal experience. As mentioned previously, watching yourself in a mirror while you learn a new movement can be a valuable experience, but unless you have a mirror next to you all the time, you will not recognize the movement outside of the place where the mirror is located. Establishing a kinesthetic sense of the action is key to improving how you move, act, and play in everyday life. By learning how to differentiate, you can create movement options that will improve the way you play and live.

A practical example of differentiation is the right-handed tennis player who habitually hits the forehand while putting most of her weight on the left leg. If the player does not quite have her legs in their habitual position to hit the forehand and instead has more weight on the right leg, she will not be able to hit the forehand with the same force and precision. Without the habitual stance, the nervous system can't recognize the body organization. With more weight on the right leg, the nervous system will be slow in figuring out which muscles should fire and in what order to execute the forehand. If, on the other hand, the player has a more flexible nervous system and has practiced the forehand with the legs in a variety of positions, it is easier for the nervous system to send the correct suggestion to the muscles and the forehand will be better timed, more powerful, and more precise.

Surely the tennis player differentiates experiences during every game. Why not just differentiate while you are performing the activity that you want to improve? Because it is difficult to differentiate while performing the activity. During an activity within a body organization such as standing, your nervous system is already firing your muscles in a specific habitual pattern, and it is difficult to stop the nervous system from firing the muscles in that pattern. So if you start differentiating the movement in the habitual position, you tend to build a movement pattern on a movement pattern. In other words, the pattern compounds rather than differentiates. However, going into an asana or position that your nervous system is not used to requires it to enter problem-solving mode and seek solutions without being already locked into the pattern of the specific activity. Then when you come back to the original position or chosen activity, the nervous system has learned something that can then be integrated into the specific activity you want to improve or change.

To return to the tennis player in the example, in order to get used to putting more weight on the left leg while doing something with the right arm, she might start doing the tree pose (see the asana exercise earlier in this chapter) first on the right leg (habitual side) while turning the upper body to the right, then on the left leg (nonhabitual side) while turning the upper body to the right. She can also do the cat and cow, putting more weight on the right side while raising the right arm toward the ceiling, and then putting more weight on the left side while raising the right arm toward the ceiling. Putting more weight on the right side while demanding action from that same side will help the nervous system recognize the movement of turning the body to the right while putting more weight on the right leg to hit the forehand. As a more advanced step, she can even hold the tennis racket in the right hand when performing the asana options. Then she can start differentiating while playing tennis.

This kind of differentiation can be done for any activity. Some people will need help with this step. It is challenging to identify what your own patterns are. You don't know what you don't know. It may be advantageous to seek input from a yoga therapist about your movement habits and patterned behaviors. For many people, identification is the most difficult step of the three. You and your yoga therapist will look at the activity you want to perform, identify what your habits are, differentiate movements in various relevant asanas based on those habits, and then integrate what has been learned into the activity that you want to improve.

Before we move on to integration, we want to clarify our view on alignment and variety of movement. It is true that there is an ideal way to perform every movement,

EXPLORATION

Differentiation

1 Perform the same movement as in the identification movement exploration. Start in a tabletop position on all fours with your knees directly under your hips and your hands directly under your shoulders.

2 Now round your spine toward the ceiling in a cat movement while your head drops to the floor.

3 On the next breath, allow your belly to sink to the floor and your head to rise toward the ceiling. Because you weren't trying to change anything, chances are you repeated this cow movement in a habitual way; you did it the same way you did before.

4 On the next breath, allow your spine to round up towards the ceiling and your head to drop towards the floor, but this time initiate the movement with the tailbone.

5 On the next breath, when your belly sinks toward the floor and your head rises towards the ceiling, begin the movement at the tailbone again.

6 The next time you repeat the cycle, begin the cat and cow movement at the head and allow movement to roll down the length of the spine.

7 This time, let the head hang down while the rest of your spine completes the cat–cow sequence.

8 Repeat the movement, but see whether you can isolate the action in the upper spine, neck, and head, keeping the lower spine still.

9 For the next few rounds, let your whole spine move, and focus on shifting your weight. What happens when you go through cat and cow pressing more firmly on the right hand? Left hand? Right knee? Left knee? How about if you focus more on the entire right side of the body? The entire left side? What happens if more weight is on the hands? When it's on the knees?

10 Try this now: As your lower spine and head lift into cow, look down. That is a different way of moving! Do the reverse so that when your spine rounds up and your head lowers, your eyes look up.

11 You can also practice differentiation through the breath. Typically, people exhale into cat and inhale into cow, so you can inhale into cat and exhale into cow instead. Reverse the breathing pattern that is normal for you. You may even try two cycles of cat–cow on the inhalation and two cycles on the exhalation. Did you increase the speed of movement or the length of breath?

12 Be creative and keep playing with cat–cow, finding new ways to initiate, breathe through, and keep the movement flowing.

13 Take a few moments to relax after challenging yourself with all those differentiated movements.

just as there is an ideal way of doing yoga asanas. Books on yoga anatomy show which muscles are engaged in each asana. What those books have not taken into account is that we are not identical. Our neurons are wired together in certain ways based on our movement habits, and not one of us will fire the muscles exactly the way it is described in the anatomy books. So while you need to think about and pay attention to alignment—what we would call an externally focused, or top-down, approach—you must also be aware of the internally focused, or bottom-up, approach. That is, what do you feel in your body? What is the right alignment for you? Not every skeleton is the same. Deviations from the norm are caused by how you developed as a child, your activity levels, and your injury histories, for example. An internalized approach will have you increase your kinesthetic intelligence by paying attention to and sensing what is right for you and your own structure so that you can adjust the asana accordingly.

Yoga can also be divided into an external or internal approach. Externally focused asana practice puts more focus on skeletal alignment, muscular engagement, balance, relaxation, and the physical sensation of a pose. Internally focused asana practice puts more focus on the mental and emotional attitudes during an asana, the ability to listen and learn from what emerges from the internal environment of the body, and an openness to all the senses. The external approach is no better or worse than the internal approach. They are different parts of the elephant. You need to have the flexibility to go back and forth between the internal and the external so that the nervous system can solve the puzzles based on not only alignment and body organization, but also on what you feel. In yoga, asanas are mind–body postures. This is a shift away from the strictly external aspects of the poses that many modern practices have embraced. As you refine skillfulness in action, you can start to perceive the skillfulness of asana based on mindful movement, not just on anatomical appearance. This means increasing awareness of habits, options, and connection through the soma. Whatever you do, when done mindfully, is an asana. To function as a synchronized whole, you need to remain stable with a steady mind no matter what external or internal puzzles emerge.

Much has been written about yoga injuries in the last few years in the daily press, research journals, and social media. It is our belief that many of the injuries are caused by focusing too much on the top-down, external approach, where the teacher adjusts the students according to some anatomical ideal while the student is in an asana, or the student strives to achieve some vision of how the "perfect" asana looks. When you differentiate, you need to pay attention to both the top-down and bottom-up approach. That is, be aware of the basic alignment of the asana, but go into the asana in a way that fits your skeleton and movement system as well as your emotions and feelings. Then play within the framework that you are comfortable with on that day. Don't do anything abrupt or too challenging when you are differentiating. Feel and sense your way to differentiation, but always remember the basic external framework of asana alignment. In the same way, don't do anything too abrupt or challenging for your internal environment either. Sense and feel how your emotions change when you differentiate an asana. Don't go further into an emotional aspect of an asana than what your nervous system can handle.

Whether you take an external or internal approach to your yoga asana practice, you are asking the nervous system to solve a puzzle. Don't make the puzzle too challenging by making the physical (balance, strength, mobility) or emotional demands too difficult. If either of those demands are too challenging, the nervous system will go back into the habitual way of doing things because the habitual way is the default position. Instead, use the Goldilocks principle when you differentiate: not too much and not too little. After the teacher sets up the framework (top-down), adapt it to your own sense of what you need right then and how much of a challenge you can handle (bottom-up). This balanced approach puts the responsibility on you, the student, to feel what is going on, increase your sensitivity to yourself, and challenge your nervous system with intelligent movement and emotional puzzles. The final step is to integrate what has been learned from identifying habits and differentiating movement during the playful asana practice.

Integration

So far, you have identified your habitual way of moving and differentiated the movement to give yourself movement options. Now it is time to integrate the differentiations of your asana or action into a synchronized whole.

In the integration phase, you allow the nervous system to incorporate what you learned during the differentiation stage. The nervous system integrated the differentiations automatically. How did this happen?

By doing asanas or any other activity in different ways, your nervous system will first receive information that the body is organized in a nonhabitual way and then send information to the muscles, making them contract in nonhabitual ways. The skeleton will move with a different timing between the joints. New internal information will be received by the brain and nervous system that will then be incorporated into your habitual way of doing the movement. It does not mean that you can't go back and perform the movement in your habitual way, but now you have options for performing the movement.

Although the idea of identification, differentiation, and integration originated in the somatic education field, similar concepts can be found in yoga. In yoga, we talk about samskaras, or imprints. In modern language, we could call those habits, which might be found in your thinking, movement, or perception. Those samskaras go through all five koshas and can shape everything you do. By identifying samskaras that prevent you from skillfully performing an activity, then differentiating your movements to promote skillful performance in different contexts and body organizations, you can finally integrate the nervous system's learning into the movement system and translate that into skillful action performed by a synchronized whole.

EXPLORATION
Integration

1 In this chapter, you have performed the cat–cow pose the habitual way, then did the asana in a multitude of different ways. Now go back and do cat–cow using your regular method. Can you feel the difference?

2 Do you notice how you are doing the cat–cow differently now compared to when you started? You are not trying to do it differently—that effort happens during the differentiation stage—but clearly you are doing the movement differently. It may be easier, larger, more coordinated, more in tune with your breathing, or altered in some other large or small way.

Importance of Renewing and Developing New Patterns

Unless you continue to play, all movements—even those that are efficient and integrated—become habitual after a while. So to continue to develop, you need to vary your asana practice and actions. Through continued playful practice, you become more sensitive to yourself and your needs. The yoga teacher or therapist sets up the framework for movement explorations, but you must take the practice off the mat.

One of the benefits of yoga in the public studio is that the teacher can help set up a safe framework for you and guide you in your practice. It is important for beginners to have class experience because everything is new. However, the more you practice yoga in a habitual, nonmindful way, the greater the risk that you will become habitual in your movements, thoughts, and actions. Options, variety, movement skills, and choices should increase with yoga practice. You should not become more rigid or stuck in your habits.

The average group yoga class consists of a lot of Simon says style of imitation. Teachers demonstrate and students mimic their poses rather than feel the asana in their own bodies and adapt. This teaching style is helpful in the beginning for visual learners. If the teacher uses undifferentiated movement patterns, it is less helpful for students, who wind up doing the asana in the way that is best for the teacher instead of for their own bodies. Meaningful movements for your own longevity must be refined from your own kinesthetic intelligence. It takes time, effort, and attention to increase this perception and responsiveness, which ultimately leads to payoff for growth, health, and movement patterns. Conversely, if you do not make the time to create variety, you won't progress long term in your skills and activities. If going to class or imitating what you did in class is all you do, then you will once again fall into a habitual movement pattern that will prevent progress in your skills and activities. The nervous system needs the juice of new puzzles.

This does not mean that you have to challenge yourself every day. Some days you need to return to familiar practice for physical, emotional, or spiritual reasons. It takes discipline (tapas) and self-study (svadhyaya) to know when to challenge the nervous system and when to let the neurons wire together a bit tighter by repeating the same movement or practice.

At some point you will hit a plateau in your skills and enthusiasm. Your movement patterns will only take you so far in a sport or in life. Yoga, with its combination of strength, mobility, and nervous system challenges, will help you develop movement pattern options that can make you more efficient and successful in your activities. You may notice that you are avoiding new situations and challenges. You have become too comfortable, and the nervous system rests and enjoys it. This is the time to mix things up and play with movement patterns again through yoga therapy. Whether or not you are an athlete, you need to challenge yourself to explore your internal and external environments so that you don't live on autopilot; rather, live life to its fullest.

Movement Habits and Injuries

Repetitive strain injuries occur frequently these days. Whether it is from office work, texting, playing tennis, running, or any other repetitive motion, modern medicine has not been able to find a way to prevent these injuries. Chapter 7 looks more specifically into a variety of injuries and how to prevent them, as well as precautions, contraindications, and ideas for rehabilitation. This section looks at repetitive injuries in general and the role habitual movement patterns might play.

Close your eyes and listen to the phrase repetitive strain injury. It sure sounds like an injury that is caused by a habitual movement. A repetitive strain injury (RSI) is caused by performing the same movement over and over again. More and more injured people are turning to yoga to deal with their aches and pains. Even though there is not a lot of research on the effectiveness of yoga for RSI, it appears that asana practice is a beneficial way to deal with these kinds of injuries.

For example, Kelly was a bank teller who found it increasingly difficult to perform the fine-motor tasks required for her job. She had become slower at sliding the coins from the counter to her palm when counting them. Bills stuck together in her fingers, or she dropped them. When she typed, her wrists and fingers seized. Kelly enjoyed how her yoga classes alleviated her back, neck, and shoulder pain and signed up for a yoga therapy session at her studio. Her yoga therapist guided her through a balanced session of basic postures, but asked her to perform them in ways she had never done before. After this session, Kelly began to play with counting money in her nondominant hand, typing with her ring fingers instead of pointer fingers, and standing on one foot while behind the counter. Gradually, she began to notice that by applying certain options, her hands performed more skillfully and the pain and seizing that was often present became less intense. Because of her yoga therapy sessions, Kelly also took a more relaxed view of the problems when they occurred.

A variety of reasons could explain why yoga is helpful with RSI. Sustained yoga practice makes people stronger, more mobile, and sensitive to how they use the body. As practice becomes established, they might also sense a need for other healthier lifestyle choices such as sleep, better food, and laughter, which contribute to injury prevention.

Another reason that yoga helps musculoskeletal and repetitive strain injuries may be that the nervous system gets to solve a problem instead of performing the same movement over and over. You learn and practice variations of the movement that caused the pain in the first place. Again, it is a process of identification, differentiation, and integration. Even though the asanas might not resemble the activity that caused the RSI, the nervous system learns something from the differentiation that it integrates into the overall movement pattern so there are options on how to move. Yoga therapy amplifies these benefits by looking at the individual's movement habits in the asanas, offering poses to deal with specific problems, and modifying the asanas to avoid irritating the injury.

Just as important in the healing of RSI is how yoga will help the overall person. It is sometimes difficult to determine what caused an RSI, but using yoga therapy and a variety of asanas increases awareness and sensitivity. It is common for a client to come in after a few yoga therapy sessions and say that she figured out that she held the breath when she did a certain repetitive movement, or that she was not present during the movement and through increased awareness has figured out what was causing the problem. It is much more empowering for clients to figure this out themselves than to have the yoga therapist or anyone else tell them. Yoga therapy is about empowerment so that the yoga therapist's guidance supports the client in discovering solutions.

In chapters 2 and 3 we provided examples of movement and asana explorations to demonstrate how you can challenge your nervous system. Chapter 4 offers more information about yoga therapy as it relates to harnessing the power of focus. Future chapters will offer instruction on creating a variety of intentional movement experiences in a yoga pose practice. All of the explorations throughout this book give you a practical understanding of the concepts of identification, differentiation, and integration so that you can improve and get more enjoyment out of asanas. They will also improve any activity in which you choose to apply these concepts from now through the course of your active lifespan!

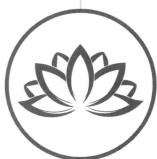

four
Developing Focus

For the last 20 years, the YogaLife Institute has taken an annual survey of the 1,000-plus yoga students who attend monthly or weekly classes there. Kristen is co-owner of the institute founded by her husband, Bob Butera, in 1996, and located in Wayne, Pennsylvania. It is a full-scale education center specializing in a holistic lifestyle approach to yoga, along with the training of yoga teachers and yoga therapists. It is also home to the Comprehensive Yoga Therapy training program, which Kristen and Staffan teach in with Bob Butera, Erin Byron, and Senior YogaLife teachers.

Questions in the annual survey are intended to solicit feedback on how we can effectively continue to serve the evolving needs of our students. Typically the survey starts by asking students for three benefits they have received from their practice. Their answers help us to better understand what motivates them to continue their yoga studies.

Every year we are delighted to see that students consistently list breath explorations as one of the top benefits they gain from practice. This is sometimes surprising when we share the survey results with our instructors, who feel like they spend the bulk of the class offering detailed instruction on the yoga poses: the transitions into the poses, refining and adapting the poses once students are in them, and the transitions out of the poses. The breath is the unifying element of all of those things, and students sense and respond to that feeling of continuity.

Although many people are familiar with yoga poses and expect them to be a part of a yoga therapy session, many people are surprised to learn that the yoga lexicon of practices extends far beyond the poses. This chapter introduces the practices of breathing, sensory mastery, visualization, and mindfulness as ways to enhance how you experience all of your life activities. Partnered with yoga poses or practiced on their own, these strategies can create a more unified experience of yoga therapy.

Yoga Therapy Beyond the Asanas

Many modern schools of yoga place a high value on the asana and physical aspects of practice. Many styles of yoga embrace this approach, and the common thread is the coordination of the poses with the breath. Of course, there are deviations from this norm, including periods of relaxation, meditation, chanting, or spiritual study and reflection.

While the types of classes that focus on asanas are pleasant and helpful for many practitioners and commonly taught, it is less common that the yoga lifestyle is taught in a group setting. The immersion into the yoga lifestyle starts with the eightfold path, which classical yoga philosophy offers as eight steps for anyone seeking enlightenment. The first two steps on this path are behavioral considerations called yamas (restraints of what is harmful) and niyamas (observances of what is pure) that guide the practitioner to consider habits to refrain from or add into their life. These considerations demonstrate one of the ways yoga therapy spills into the activities associated with daily life.

The purpose of the eightfold path is to connect people with the wisdom of the ages, while soliciting introspection, contemplation, stability of the body, freedom of the breath, sensory mastery, stillness of mind, spiritual awakening, and ultimately, self-realization. The eightfold path is a book unto itself; so for our purpose of supporting the active lifestyle, we will focus on four practical, immediately applicable practices that can be explored on their own or in tandem with yoga poses: breathing, sensory mastery, visualization, and mindfulness.

Power of the Breath

Breath is central to who we are. Whether it relates to our ability to work, think, sleep, or interact with others, we might claim that the breath is the core pattern that drives all other patterns. After all, what other activity do we perform six to eight million times per year? Adapting the breath helps people change along with life. Learning to consciously engage with the breath enables people to tap into a central part of themselves.

Superficial breathing ensures a superficial experience of ourselves.

—The Tao of Natural Breathing, Dennis Lewis

History is full of examples of cultures connecting breath, soul, and spirit in one way or another. The Bible states that God breathed life into Adam. The Hindus spoke about *atman*. The Greeks spoke about *pneuma*. The Romans spoke about *spiritus*. The Hebrews spoke about *ruach*. The Chinese spoke about *chi* or *qi*. In Hawaii, outsiders were called *haoles*, translating to no breath or breathless.

In yoga we have the concept of prana, which is often translated as life force, energy, or vitality and is connected with the fourth step on the eightfold path, pranayama. Pranayama is often translated as breath control or breath mastery. We like to think of pranayama more in terms of breathing skills in general, primarily being able to use the breath as a resource for self-awareness and working from that awareness, the ability to adapt the breath to the situation. To explore that self-awareness through the breath, you have to identify, differentiate, and integrate your breath just like you do with any other movement.

How you breathe at any given time can enhance or detract from what you are trying to accomplish. Although most of the time breathing is an involuntary act, we can be mindful and skillful enough to make it a voluntary act. Chances are if you have never done breathing practices before, you will be shocked by how they effect immediate changes in your life experience. At first, it might be challenging to cultivate the attention needed to notice these changes; be patient as you explore. To become a skillful breather, you may first have to uncover and remove the obstacles between yourself and a free, adaptable breath. To do this, you need to go through a familiar process with your current breathing patterns.

To become a skillful breather, follow this process:

1. Cultivate the discipline to observe your existing breathing habits (identification).
2. Introduce new options (differentiation).
3. Adapt your breath to support and enhance all of your activities (integration).

As you start the breathing exercises, remember that having options implies that you don't do things in the same way over and over. Your nervous system will not become adaptable if you replicate a breath exploration or any other exploration without variety. The term exploration implies variation. Once you start to explore more options for breathing, it will become challenging at times to identify whether you are, in fact, doing what you think you are doing. As you explore, try to stay curious and playful. If you notice that you are creating unnecessary strain or tension in your body, stop the exercise, pause for a few moments to notice, and then start again with an attitude of curiosity and playfulness.

The positional breath exploration offers you the chance to adapt your breath to various positions. In this breath exploration, depending on your orientation and how well you are able to perceive your breath, you may be able to notice differences in how you breathe. Observe, play, and have fun!

The positional breath exploration also offers you the opportunity to understand a foundational understanding of how you engage with your breath and starts the process of making your breathing a more conscious act. The awareness that you gather from this exercise gives you a baseline understanding from which to begin to differentiate your breath and develop new breathing options.

Options in breathing or movements imply a freedom to choose. The freedom to choose is a joyful activity for the development of the nervous system. Observe a child with a new coloring book. He plays and experiments with coloring methods: different crayon strokes and pressures, holding the crayons in either hand or between various fingers or in a fist. He may initiate the movement from his small knuckles, wrists, or elbows, or he may use the entire arm to make sweeping scribbles across the page. There appears to be no method or reason in how he colors and you think that you could probably teach the child to make a prettier, cleaner work without all the randomness and inevitable mess. However, the child's nervous system is learning all the variations that are needed to understand how to work with the crayons in the future: how to create different shades and textures based on movement and pressure, how to color within the lines, and how to get the desired effect from his hands with the rest of the body in various postures, with the head perched in diverse positions, and with all kinds of distractions going on inside and outside. In short, the nervous system is learning options through free experimentation so that the child can color in all kinds of ways.

This kind of freedom is also required of the breath if we are to navigate different life situations and experiences. Once you start playing with breathing patterns in various combinations, you will notice that after the differentiations are integrated, the nervous system will choose the pattern that is the most efficient for a particular circumstance in the moment. In other words, by experimenting with your options for breathing, you can choose the one that best fits the situation. The better you can adapt your breath to different situations, the better you will be able to function in all kinds of situations. Differentiating breathing patterns gives the nervous system options so that you can respond to life effectively.

Positional Breath

❶ Start in a reclined position on the floor, on a yoga mat, or on any firm surface that will provide tactile feedback about how your body is resting on the floor. Observe your breath without changing it. Be curious and don't judge yourself.

❷ Where does your breath originate from? In the abdomen? Chest? Collarbones?

❸ Does your abdomen move up and out toward the ceiling as well as back and down into the floor?

❹ Does the rib cage move up and out toward the ceiling as well as back and down into the floor?

❺ Put your hands on the side of your body at your lower ribs (a). Can you feel expansion into your hands?

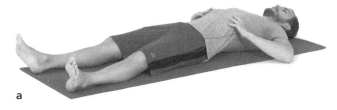

a

❻ Can you feel the sides of your rib cage expand? If not, can you expand your breath sideways, making your rib cage expand?

❼ As you're doing this, notice whether the left side of the rib cage expands in the same way as the right side of the rib cage.

❽ Where do you feel muscular contraction when you breathe out?

❾ Roll over facedown, crossing your arms and allowing your forehead to rest on them (b). Now repeat the same observations that you made in the reclined position. How does the feedback change? Can you feel the expansion in the back of the torso a little more? Can you use the floor to give you more feedback about what is happening in the front of the body in the abdomen and rib cage?

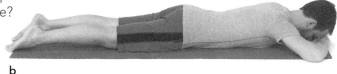

b

❿ Come up to standing (c), paying attention to how you use your breath in the transition from facedown to upright. Did you use your breath or did you hold it? Now repeat the same observations that you did in the other two positions. Where do you feel expansion when you breathe in? Where do you feel contraction when you breathe out? How did your perception of your breath change when you were standing? Was it more difficult for you to feel your breath without the floor to give you feedback?

⓫ Are you able to perceive that each change of position changes your potential experience of your breath? Acknowledge the breathing habits present in each of the positions.

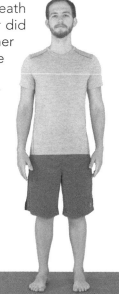

c

Breathing and Stress Reduction

The breath is unique in that it can change how you feel, regulate the balance between the sympathetic (SNS) and parasympathetic nervous systems (PNS), and make you feel stressed or relaxed. It is all within your control. Many other autonomic functions central to survival such as heart rate, function of the internal organs, and blood pressure are not within conscious control, but breathing is. Maybe that is why so many traditions have emphasized breathing and connected the breath to the soul, spirit, life force, and vitality.

In general, one can say that by slowing the breath, the PNS has a dampening effect on the SNS. You become less stressed, heart rate goes down, and food is absorbed more efficiently. You enter a state in which healing can take place. On the other hand, if you breathe faster, the SNS comes roaring back and you are back into "fight, flight, or freeze" mode. When you are anxious, you also tend to breathe more shallowly and at a faster rate. Do you know how your breath changes when you are stressed? Does the breath change before you realize that you are stressed?

The breathing for stress and relaxation exercise helps you wake up your whole torso—that is abdomen, chest, and clavicles—during the breath. Depending on how you perform this breath, it can have a relaxing PNS response or energizing SNS response. It depends on how you perform the exercise and how your mind interprets what you are doing. Even though most of us need more PNS activation, we have to be aware that depending on the state we are in and how we perform the exploration, it can have an energizing or calming effect on us. For the next breath exploration, you will first observe your normal breath, introduce new options to your breathing, and then go back to observing the breath to assess how the new information is being integrated.

The breathing for stress and relaxation exercise also gives you a chance to get to know which breathing pattern makes you feel more relaxed or stressed. Pay attention to how you feel both physically and emotionally during breath explorations. While explorations during asana practice can evoke emotions, exploring the breath without attaching movement to it can be even more emotional for some people. It is important that you notice what happens when you explore or play with the breath and notice what your reactions are to breath or asana explorations.

When working with the breath, not everyone reacts the same. There is no universal response to breathing practices. Pay attention to how you feel physically, emotionally, and mentally during breath explorations. Because breath is central to who we are at our deepest core (literally and metaphysically), it is normal and healthy to experience a variety of reactions when playing with your breathing patterns. Many outgrowths associated with a breathing practice will be pleasant, but it is also possible that mucking around with your breathing habits will be slightly unpleasant. Playing with the breath might shine a light of awareness on aspects of yourself that were previously hidden or suppressed. Both comfortable and uncomfortable outcomes are normal; you may even experience some of both.

I (Staffan) once spoke to a friend who was trying to meditate, who told me that every time she tried to meditate she became more anxious. She could not figure out why it was happening because she believed that meditation was supposed to calm her down. After dialogue and observation, we realized that her breathing patterns were making her anxious. Her meditation teacher always started the sessions with the suggestion to breathe deeply without offering specific instructions for what that

Breathing for Stress and Relaxation

1 Start in a reclined position on the floor, on a yoga mat, or on any firm surface that will give you tactile feedback about how your body is resting on the floor.

2 Exaggerate the movement of your abdomen rising as you breathe in and exaggerate pulling the abdomen in as you breathe out. How does that feel? This is what many people consider normal, diaphragmatic breathing. (It is interesting to note that no air enters the abdomen even though it may feel or appear that way. The rising of the abdomen is a function of the diaphragm, one of your primary breathing muscles, descending and displacing the organs in the abdomen. All breathing is diaphragmatic unless you are incapacitated in some way.)

3 Go back to your normal breathing pattern. Notice a difference? Make note of what you observed.

4 What happens in your rib cage and chest when you allow the diaphragm to move more freely? Can you exaggerate the movement of your rib cage as you breathe in and out? Can you allow your rib cage to collapse as the abdomen expands when you breathe in? Can you expand your rib cage and pull your abdomen in as you breathe out? How does that feel? Can you keep your rib cage absolutely still as you allow your abdomen to expand and pull back in?

5 Go back to your normal breathing pattern. Notice a difference? Make note of what you observed.

6 Now reverse the movement of the rib cage and the abdomen. Allow your rib cage to expand and your abdomen to pull in as you breathe in, and then collapse the rib cage and expand the abdomen as you breathe out. This is called reverse breathing and is frequently used in martial arts or when people expect to use a lot of effort. You don't want to breathe in a reversed fashion during everyday activities, but when you need to use maximum effort it can be important to be able to reverse breathe.

7 Go back to your normal breathing pattern. Notice a difference? Make note of what you observed.

8 Now put your fingers above and behind the collarbones, or clavicles. Can you feel movement there when you breathe? Can you gently increase the movement there as you breathe in? Can you feel your abdomen pull in as you increase the movement in the upper part of the lungs? How do you feel? Anxious? Most people will feel anxious when they breathe more from the area around the clavicles. The muscles in that area are much smaller and are normally only used when you need a large effort, or when you are anxious. Sometimes these muscles activate when a person has a condition that prevents the use of the diaphragm or decreases lung capacity.

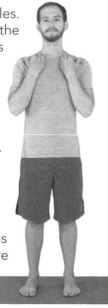

9 Now resume your normal breathing pattern. What did you do to relieve the anxiety? Did you go back to belly breathing? Did you slow your breath? How has your breathing changed since you started this exploration?

10 Stand up. How do you feel standing now compared to the previous exercise when you noticed your standing breath? Do you feel more aware of your breath? Can you perform some of the alternative ways of breathing while standing?

actually meant. My friend's interpretation of breathe deeply was to breathe into her upper chest, which was making her anxious. Once we changed the intention to breathe slowly and explored the possibilities associated with that intention, the anxiety subsided and she began to enjoy meditation.

Be aware that some practices will work well most of the time, while others might only be helpful at the right time in your life. Only you know whether you are challenging yourself at the appropriate level at the right time. If you are unsure of an exploration, back off for a while and revisit it later to see whether you get the same results. It is important to be responsive to your experiences and give yourself permission to adapt and refine the practices according to your own intentions and ability to engage at any given time. What might have been a useful exploration at one time might not be useful in future situations. You might have changed and don't need that specific practice any longer. Don't hold onto what is not useful. Move on to new explorations.

Different styles of yoga use the breath to create distinct results. Practitioners of some styles have specific ideas about what they believe correct breathing is. We have noticed that many experienced yoga practitioners have rigid breathing habits. What comes to light after they work with breath explorations for a while is that they had not identified their existing breathing patterns when they started practicing yoga. Instead they adopted what they believed to be the "yogic" breathing pattern, and in doing so, layered a new pattern on top of an old one. This is just one example of how differentiation without identification is less effective when the desired outcome is freedom and flexibility of the breath. To be truly adaptable, you must identify your starting point and then create options.

You will notice that in considering options, we tend to stay away from words such as right, correct, controlled, and superior and other value judgments about breathing practices. Instead, we aim to inspire you to consider the many ways that you can explore how to remove the patterns that interfere with your free, easy, and adaptable breath. The explorations we have outlined so far are not exhaustive, but they do give you a good sense of what is possible when you bring an attitude of curiosity and exploration to breathing. As you play with breath, it is our preference that in this stage you favor building a sense of observation, adaptability, and responsiveness over the idea of superimposing a pattern, controlling the breath, or even breathing "correctly." We encourage you to stay interested in using the breath explorations as a way to discover options that are best suited to the activity that you want to perform.

So far you have identified how you are breathing and explored various differentiations for your breath, and then you paid attention to how the differentiations were integrated into your normal breath pattern. Having done the basic identification, differentiation, and integration, you can now continue to work on integrating the differentiations into your daily activities.

We will revisit the breath in other chapters and offer you additional breathing options you can explore in tandem with various yoga poses. For now, we will move on to playing with the sense-mastery (pratyahara) limb of the eightfold path.

Sensory Awareness

The fifth step in the eightfold path of yoga is pratyahara, which is often translated as sense mastery or sensory withdrawal. Pratyahara is considered to be the bridge between the external petals of yoga (yamas, niyamas, asana, and pranayama) and the internal petals of yoga (dharana, dhyana, and samadhi).

After all the emphasis we have put on paying attention to sensations in order to identify, differentiate, and integrate, it might sound strange that we now suggest that you attempt to work on withdrawing the senses. It is true that for yoga therapy practices to be more personalized and effective, you need to refine all of your senses as a way to better understand and respond to yourself and the world around you. But it is also true that yoga therapy will be more effective if you eliminate unwelcomed sensory distractions. So far we have played with refining your senses by guiding you to tune into obvious sensations (and maybe some not-so-obvious ones!) via targeted explorations. In this section, we will train our senses to focus where we want them and disregard what we don't need to attend to.

Although sensory input isn't always under your control, you can control how you respond to your senses. You can actually choose where to focus your attention. Think of a time you were so engrossed in an activity that you did not hear someone speaking to you. This level of attention is an example of how sense mastery works. You are able to completely attend to what is important and selectively disregard other input. The practice of sensory withdrawal is an excellent way to avoid distractions so that you can focus all of your energy into the activity at hand.

Let's go back to our tennis player to explore how the practice of pratyahara might help her improve her game. To harness attention, the tennis player might focus on using one sense at a time, for example listening to the sound of the ball, the vibrations of the hand as the racket makes contact, or listening to the breath as a way of tuning out noise from fellow players or spectators. By focusing on one area, the tennis player can avoid being distracted by internal or external factors that will hinder her ability to focus on the game.

As you can see from the tennis example, pratyahara can be practiced in many ways and the focus can be either internal or external. Let's start with using the breath as a point of focus in the following exercise.

This exercise combines the practices of breathing (pranayama) and sense mastery (pratyahara). By attuning to your breath and linking the breath with various activities, you continue to challenge your ability to focus and tune out distractions. Please note that while you are tuning out distractions when you are practicing pratyahara,

EXPLORATION

Pratyahara Breath

1 Sit in a chair. Make sure your spine is upright and that you are not slouching against the back of the chair. Close your eyes.

2 Feel how the air is coming in through your nostrils. How far down the throat or into the lungs can you feel the incoming air? As you breathe out, can you feel the air emptying out of your lungs, all the way through your nose or mouth?

3 Complete 10 breath cycles (inhale and exhale), paying attention to the air coming into and leaving your lungs.

4 Open your eyes for 10 breath cycles. Now that your vision is available to you, is it easier or more difficult to pay attention to the air coming and going?

5 Stand up and walk around the room, still paying attention to the breath coming and going. Does that make it easier or more difficult to pay attention to your sense of breath in the lungs?

you are at the same time increasing your awareness of your surroundings by being mindful. You are learning how to tune out information in your environment that is distracting.

Using sensory withdrawal in daily life activities produces amazing benefits, especially in the current climate of unlimited distractions. Most of us are constantly on; smart phones enable us to check e-mail, text, and search the Web for news, sport scores, and whatever else we want to know anytime. The amount of information we consume in combination with the level of multitasking required for us to sort and process it is overwhelming at times, and our experience and enjoyment of many activities are suffering because of it.

We are often distracted by the simple fact that we *can* check all of this information whenever we want to. Every time we get a new text, Facebook like, or similar electronic attention, a small surge of feel-good dopamine enters the brain. Maybe your own phone is on your desk or in your pocket while you are working so you can check it regularly. Does it ever "call your name"? Today many people experience phantom buzzing from their phones, thinking it vibrated when it didn't. This phenomenon is the nervous system looking for an easy ping of dopamine. We set up this biological reward system based on our patterns of interacting with our electronic gadgets, and as a result we are more distracted than ever.

Can you stop yourself from checking your smartphone? When you are working at your computer how often do you check e-mail? When you are out with friends or at the dinner table with your family, do you have the urge to check your phone? It is easy for many of us to be distracted by our electronic gadgets. The next time you are out in a public space like a mall, park, downtown area, or train station, take a few minutes to notice how many people are distracted by their electronics. Many people do not notice what they are missing around them because they are distracted by technology in some way.

Pratyahara limits the pull of electronics and other distractions. From a daily-life perspective, practicing sense mastery allows you to withdraw from, selectively attend to, or ignore all those sensory temptations. That way, you can focus on a specific activity or goal. The next exercise explores how you can focus on a specific sound in your environment as a way to harness your sense mastery.

EXPLORATION
Pratyahara Sound

1 Go for a run or a walk without electronics or headphones. Listen to the sound of your feet hitting the ground. Does it sound the same when the left foot hits the ground as when the right foot hits the ground? Can you change the sound? Can you make the sound softer? Louder?

2 Challenge yourself to ignore all the other sounds and visual input around you and just listen to the repetitive sound of your feet hitting the ground.

3 Once you have played with several sounds of your feet hitting the ground, go back to your normal stride. Did the sound change from when you started the exploration?

Did you realize that during this exercise you once again applied the concepts of identification, differentiation, and integration? The only shift from the movement variations of the previous chapter was that you paid attention to a sound instead of an action.

You can also use pratyahara to focus on a specific body part. Instead of focusing on the *sound* the feet make hitting the ground, a runner could focus on the *way* the feet hit the ground. The tennis player could focus on a forearm and wrist connection to the racket and ball. You can pay attention to any body part, but initially it is probably more relevant to pay attention to a part of the body that is most involved in the activity that you are doing. This helps you customize your approach and subsequently focus on increasingly subtle aspects of your body. The following exercise gives you the opportunity to practice this body awareness and customization.

This pratyahara activity gives you the chance to gain sense mastery over a longer period of time. You can see how selective attention improves your movement abilities as well.

Pratyahara can also be a helpful tool to support your yoga pose and meditation practices. In tree pose you might pay attention to the foot that you balance on or your breath or set your eyes on a singular focal point. When you are practicing practical pratyahara, you are trying to focus on one thing without being disturbed by anything else that your senses pick up. These potential disturbances may include your smartphone, family, pets, yoga teacher, or what is happening outside the window.

EXPLORATION
Pratyahara Body

1 Pick one of your favorite activities and select a body part to focus on. Anchor your attention to this body part during the activity every time you practice it.

2 Perform the activity while focusing on the particular body part for a specific period of time (depending on the frequency of the activity, we suggest three to four weeks). During that time you may note small insights about things you have identified, differentiated, and perhaps even integrated.

3 At the end of the designated time, assess what you have learned through this exercise.

Visualization

Visualization is a powerful sensory tool that lends itself to yoga pose practice. Common yoga language includes words such root, flow, ground, open, lengthen, blossom, fly, reach, and spread, which all have rich visual associations. The names of yoga poses (warrior, lion, tree, crescent moon, goddess, hero, and mountain to mention a few) are loaded with powerful images for the practitioner to embody. For people who have the ability to think visually, partnering a visualization practice with your chosen activity can at the very least enhance the experience, and for some, it can dramatically change the outcome of the action or yoga posture.

Let's go back to our friend the tennis player. She might visualize external results such as acing a serve, the ball slicing away from her opponent, the scoreboard changing in her favor, or simply seeing herself winning the match. Conversely, the tennis player might internalize a visual image associated with a particular quality, like being graceful as a gazelle, fluid as a dancer, or focused like a Zen master.

The following exercise calls on your internal visual sense. Notice the power that visualization has over your ability to perform an activity.

EXPLORATION

Visualization

1 Stand in mountain pose. (See chapter 2 for basic mountain pose instructions.)

2 How do you feel "just standing here"? Make note of what you notice.

3 What happens when you change the intention from "I am just standing here" to "I am in mountain pose"?

4 Now visualize a mountain. Create an image in your mind of a strong, rocky body rising out of the earth's crust up into the clouds. What happens when you do that? Do you feel heavy? Light? Grounded? Do you feel a shift in the way you embody the pose?

5 Now visualize the base of the mountain—firm, unyielding, and strong. Do you feel a shift in the way you embody the pose?

6 Now visualize lava erupting from the top of the mountain in hot, red plumes. What happens to your attention? Did it shift to a different area of the body? What happened to your mind when the lava erupted? Did you feel more or less settled when the lava erupted?

7 Go back to "just standing here" and see what differences you notice in your posture. Make note of what you observe.

Mountain pose is just one of many poses that can be enhanced by practicing visualization. Yoga poses can also be divided into archetypes. For example, downward dog is an animal archetype. When you do downward dog what do you visualize? Do you visualize a playful dog? A sleepy dog just waking itself up? Hopefully it's not an angry dog. Or maybe you just do the downward dog and feel a great stretch in the back of your legs and back. That is okay too, but every now and then you can play with visualization to create a different experience.

By now you are probably sensing that we will not tell you what you should be doing in your yoga practice. Instead, we offer options that you can engage with as they become interesting or relevant. It is up to you to connect these choices to the activities that you intend to enhance using yoga therapy. The question each time you come to your mat can be "How do I want to practice today? What is my intention?" Some days it might be for a stretching sensation. Other days you might go for a sense of strength or endurance, and on other days you might work on withdrawing your senses, internalizing your attention, or applying visualization or mindfulness techniques. All of these options are appropriate when the right practitioner does them with conscious awareness at the right time. The important thing is that you are empowered to tailor your practice to your needs in the moment so that you don't get stuck in one specific visualization, breath pattern, or intention for your practice.

For our part, we suggest that you avoid focusing on too many things at the same time. By the end of this book, you will have learned at least 32 poses with many variations attached to each one. You may become so excited about learning these things that you want to do them all at once. It's a normal reaction. If that happens, it's important to remember that one of the benefits of setting a clear intention is its singular focus. Recall how in chapter 1 we talked about how we are all negatively affected by doing too many things at once? Try giving yourself the luxury of focusing on one or two things at a time in your practice. Too many intentions or areas of focus can muddy the waters and render practices less effective. We will further explore the many possibilities of intention in practice in chapter 8.

In chapter 3 we discussed that somatic educators operate under the assumption that each state of mind has a corresponding body organization. If we hold that assumption to be true, then that also means that each body organization has a corresponding state of mind. Your mental state is reflected in the body and vice versa. Change your mind and your body will change, or change your body and your mind will change. As a refresher, you might want to do the body language exploration in chapter 3.

Regardless of how you choose to go about it, yoga therapy offers intelligent approaches to effect change in the body and mind. These shifts allow you to verify and understand the infinite connections and interrelationships between your body and mind.

The benefit of visualization is not a new discovery. Visualization has been employed in some way or other by a variety of physical and spiritual disciplines throughout the ages. In both ancient and modern times, many high-level athletes have used visualization; it has often been said that you can't win an Olympic medal without visualizing yourself winning it. If you watch great athletes step onto the court, pitch, rink, or any other athletic arena, they carry themselves in a certain way. They are grounded and they have an aura around them that says "I am good."

Take a moment to consider this for yourself. How do you carry yourself when you are approaching a new activity or task? Do you carry yourself with the belief that you will be able to accomplish it or that you are unlikely to accomplish the task? Does the way you carry yourself shape your attitude? Does the way you organize your body sabotage your change of success in your chosen task? More than likely if you visualize yourself failing, you will!

This next exercise gives you the opportunity to apply the power of visualization to your own experience. Notice what happens when you differentiate your mental images.

EXPLORATION
Visualization of Personal Performance

1 Lie on the floor. Make yourself comfortable and close your eyes.

2 Think of an activity that you would like to do or an activity that you would like to perform better. Visualize yourself being successful at the activity. How do you feel when you are successful in the activity? How does your sense of yourself change? Which muscles do you tighten so that they are ready to spring to action?

3 Now visualize yourself being unsuccessful in the same activity. How do you feel this time? How does your body organize itself when you don't do well in the activity?

4 Come up to standing. Are you able to visualize yourself being successful in the activity again? Can you now go back and forth between visualizing yourself being successful and failing? What differences do you sense in how your body organizes itself between those two states?

Apply the insights from the previous exercise. Now that you can sense the difference in how you organize your body in each of those states, use the successful body organization. Next time you go to perform the activity, visualize yourself being successful before you practice it. Be aware of when the body starts going into the organization where you are not successful. Notice when that happens and visualize a successful outcome again.

You can visualize yourself doing something in two ways. One is to visualize from inside yourself and the other is to visualize from outside yourself. Let's say you are running a race. You spend a few minutes before the race visualizing yourself being successful. Some people visualize themselves from the inside. That is, they cannot see themselves, but they can see the competitors next to them, their surroundings, and the road. Another person might see himself running the course as if watching a movie. He is visualizing himself from the outside. No research has determined whether one way is better than the other.

What does seem clear is that the more senses you include when you visualize, the more effective it is. Runners in the example may incorporate the sounds of the crowd or their feet hitting the ground. They can incorporate the kinesthetic sense of running and the breath in their lungs and the smell of the air. We started this section by visualizing mountain pose, so let us return to the mountain for this visualization exercise.

By differentiating your imagined senses and experimenting with visualization, you fortify your ability to act in varied and efficient ways. Pratyahara requires you to filter external sensory input as well as apply internal sensory input in masterful ways. Thus, you gain greater control over your internal and, by extension, external realms.

EXPLORATION
Multiple-Sense

1 Stand in mountain pose. Visualize yourself as a mountain.

2 Add other senses into this visualization. What sounds are there? Smells? Movements? Tastes? Let it come to you through all of your senses.

3 Now let the volcano inside the mountain explode again. How did the senses change? How can you use the senses to pull you back to the original mountain pose?

Bhava or Mental Attitudes

Bhava, state of body and mind, or attitude, is a yogic concept related to the interrelationship between your body and mind. Bhava influences how you experience a pose, your posture, your mood, and other factors. Attitudes are the foundational underpinning of all yoga poses; in fact, one definition of the pose is to assume a particular attitude or position. The four main categories of bhavas are dharma (duty), jnana (knowledge), vairagya (nonattachment), and aiswarya (self-reliance or mastery). You can play with the bhavas in several ways.

You can do an asana or activity and see which attitude you experience. What is important is that you experience the bhava as it is, not the attitude you felt yesterday or what you expect to feel. You might think that you should feel the attitude of knowledge if you sit down and try to write something (like we do right now as we are writing this book), but depending on what you write, you might feel something different. You might experience the attitude of duty to write a thank you note, or mastery to write a manual on how to build something. The important thing is that you pay attention to your experience of the present bhava as you are performing the activity.

You can do an asana or activity, observe the attitude you experience today, and then change the attitude. Visualization may be helpful. You can either sense in your body how it would feel to have a certain attitude or you can visualize it. Play with both. Some of you will do better with sensing the attitude kinesthetically while others will do better visualizing the attitude.

You can also visualize or sense an attitude before you enter the asana. When people practice asana they often forget about the transition between postures and aren't aware of how to go into and out of them. Assuming an attitude before you go into an asana or sequence helps you maintain that attitude throughout the routine of entering, maintaining, and exiting the asana. The following exercise gives you the opportunity to experience this.

EXPLORATION
Bhava Visualization

1 In this exploration you will transition from the mountain pose (chapter 2) into the standing forward fold. Pause to notice what your attitude is before you get into the pose.

2 Start in mountain pose. Is your mind quiet here or are you thinking about how to get into your standing forward fold?

3 Fold forward. How did you get there? Did your attitude change on the way down?

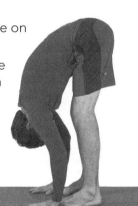

4 Hold the forward fold. What do you feel? Did your attitude change? Did you allow yourself to sense which bhava emerged when you entered the asana, or had you already decided what attitude you would have?

5 Try it again. Go back to mountain pose and then enter into the forward fold. Did you sense the same attitude?

6 Stay in the forward fold. Try out four attitudes by visualizing them: strength, freedom, openness, and surrender. Can you feel the subtle change in body organization that occurs when you visualize and shift into a different attitude?

7 Come up with and visualize another bhava that you would like to explore. How does that shift the organization of your body in both poses?

8 Perform the mountain pose to forward fold combination with the intention of sensing the attitudes as they emerge rather than superimposing an attitude onto the sequence.

Again, with this exercise we applied our basic concepts of identification, differentiation, and integration. You sensed which initial attitude emerged, then you embodied and visualized four different attitudes, integrated, and allowed a final—possibly new—attitude to come through. In the previous movement exploration, visualization helped you find the body organization that corresponded to each attitude, and then at the end, the body was able to integrate all four of the attitudes and choose the attitude that felt right at the time. Why do you have to visualize each attitude? Wasn't it clear that your body picked the most appropriate attitude to start with? That is only true if you can organize your body in a way that allows you to experience each attitude. Visualization can help you find different, hard-to-reach organizations of your body that will then allow you to experience each attitude within you.

If we go back to the idea that each emotional state has a corresponding body organization, and that each body organization has a corresponding emotional state, then it follows that if you cannot organize your body in a certain way, you will not be able to reach that emotional state or attitude. New research also seems to indicate that the way people hold their bodies affects how they feel and act. So how does this relate to the activity or movement that you want to perform?

Mindfulness

The concept of mindfulness is applied to many fields of study these days: health care, business, education, meditation, weight loss, and so on. Here we apply mindfulness to the process of improving movement and staying active throughout life. Mindfulness is the ability to observe one's thoughts, emotions, actions, and experiences from moment to moment with nonjudgmental awareness.

The "moment to moment" part is important for yoga therapy practice. Mindfulness requires being present, not thinking about the future or the past. Because you have played with the movement explorations in this book, you are already on your way toward practicing mindfulness. To identify, differentiate, and integrate, you need to mindfully stay in the present moment and observe yourself without judging your movements, actions, and thoughts as good or bad. Because as soon as you judge, you have compared the movement to something else and left the present moment behind. Just observe yourself neutrally. Sounds simple, right . . . or not?

Mindfulness requires patience, willingness for self-study (svadhyaya), and time and space for reflection. Mindfulness does not require the *why* of your actions. Why you do something might lead you down a trail that never ends and into the past or the future. As soon as you start thinking about improving the movement, you might start thinking about biomechanics or anatomy and stop sensing how you are doing something.

Instead of judgment or analysis, mindfulness is about observing the *how*. Not questioning the how but just a simple "How do I do what I do?" How am I acting in the world toward others, toward myself? How do I do that movement or action? Just how: curiosity, sensing, feeling! Insights into the *why* might emerge, but what is important is how you do something. Until you know the how, you can't change what you are doing.

The first step toward mindfulness is to identify what you are doing. Then stop, pause, and decide to go ahead and do it mindfully, or differentiate and decide to do something else. The important thing is that you did not perform the action automatically. After you pause the action enough times to develop options based on the context you are in, you will integrate the mindful behavior into every behavior. Even mindfulness comes back to identify, differentiate, and integrate.

Remember the quote by Moshe Feldenkrais from the previous chapter: "*If you don't know what you are doing, you can't do what you want.*" How do you know what you are doing? By being mindful of your actions and movements! Up until this point in the book, everything that we have discussed has been about mindfulness and self-study: How do you do what you do? Every exploration so far falls under the umbrella of mindfulness; they were all anchored in observing yourself in the present moment. Asana is how you move in the present—not in the past or future. Pranayama is about breathing in the present. Pratyahara is about being present and able to focus the senses. It's about mastering both external and internal senses until you can eventually reach a state of oneness and bliss.

In the section on visualization, you became aware of present attitudes or bhavas. Mindfulness is simply awareness in the present! Of course, staying present may be one of the most difficult things to do in modern life. There is work to be done, people to take care of, e-mail to attend to, books to read, learning to do. It is challenging to stay present.

Tying These Concepts Together and Applying Them to Life

The great news is that once the yoga therapy practice and lifestyle take hold, you can apply what you learn in your practice to your daily life. You can meditate while in the bathtub or cooking dinner, choose healthy movements while doing the dishes, embrace an attitude of joy while playing tennis, be more focused at work, feel more compassionate toward yourself and others, and yes, even mindfully use your technology.

Yoga unites the past and the future by bringing you into the present. In the present moment, there is no ideal to live up to. We truly believe that mindfully practicing yoga can take you to a place where you are completely aware in the moment, able to take on challenges, and be curious about the world without getting caught up in it.

The yoga practices that we present in the rest of this book are a small sliver of what yoga therapy has to offer. We have narrowed our intention in order to help you apply basic principles of yoga therapy to support your active lifestyle. The practices we present all require mindfulness. That is, they require you to be fully present and in the moment and ask you to be aware of how you are doing what you are doing without judgment.

Be mindful when you are doing the poses with small variations, when you are getting in and out of poses in different ways, when you are changing attitudes, when you breathe, when you withdraw your senses, and when you visualize. By playing with and varying all these factors, letting them float in and out of the foreground of your practice, you will give yourself options in life. Your goal is not to remove habits that get in the way of more efficient actions. But because you will have different options, you can free yourself from having to use those habits when they are inefficient. By learning to focus on one aspect or another during your asana practice, you will find that you will become more focused in your actions off the yoga mat.

Yoga's concept of mindfulness is related to the concept of flow, or zone consciousness, and is used as a basis for further explorations of different physical fitness activities in later chapters. Mihaly Csikszentmihalyi wrote the book *Flow: The Psychology of Optimal Experience* in 1990. Flow is defined as a mental state in which the person is fully immersed in the activity he or she is performing. The person performing the activity is enjoying the process and is fully absorbed and single minded in what he or she does. Flow can be experienced in many activities and is sometimes described as being in the zone.

One often hears about athletes being in the zone. This phenomenon also happens when chefs cook and parents interact with children and in many other activities. Time slows and it seems like anything is possible. One can do no wrong. Then the next day it is gone. We look for the zone, but the more we look, the less likely we are to find it. In flow, everything is aligned and focused. It can happen in an asana practice when the mindfulness, breath, movement, attitude, focus, and intention are all aligned. This goes beyond just simple movement; the zone suggests a complete focus and immersion in the activity being performed. The person is in the present.

With focused practice using the principles outlined so far, we believe that it is possible that on some days you will catch a glimpse of flow, the zone, or a complete mindfulness state. Whether you do that or not depends on how motivated you are to apply the principles of this book to your practice and life. To stay active throughout your life, you need to apply these principles to the activities that you want to enjoy from now on. The more you apply what you are learning here, and on and off of your yoga mat, the more you will be able to enjoy a long, healthy, active life.

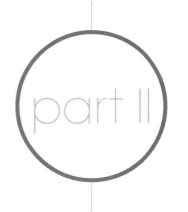

Foundations of
Practice

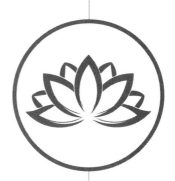

five
Basic Practices and Props

People come in different shapes, sizes, colors, and dispositions and have different gifts and nuanced ways of interacting with the world. This variety isn't unique to being human. Variability exists among all living organisms and the ecological systems in which they reside. The next time you are someplace where lots of people are walking around—the mall, beach, park, or downtown area—take a moment to sit and observe how many sizes and shapes of bodies pass by. Then look at how they walk. From where do they initiate the walking action? How much effort or ease do they bring to the act of walking? What position is their head in relative to the spine? Do they have a dominant leg or foot? How are their hips and pelvis moving? Which part of their foot hits the ground first? Do they do the same thing with each foot?

You don't have to be a movement expert to be able to see the similarities between people during the act of walking—in most cases, one foot in front of the other—yet the details of how each person walks varies greatly. If you were to transfer the same powers of observation to an activity such as tennis, swimming, or golf, you would notice similarities and differences in how people perform those activities as well.

The same thing applies to yoga pose practices. No two people experience a yoga pose in exactly the same way, nor should they strive to. Range of motion in the joints and muscle activations differ depending on bone structure, lifestyle habits, emotional responses, previous training, past injuries, and a person's conscious or unconscious intention for practice.

Anatomy books offer great insight into the body, but they often present us with an illusion that there is a standard body, when the reality is that the person depicted in the book represents an average that doesn't actually exist. Although we all might have the same parts, how those parts are made and then function together can vary dramatically from person to person. This average is necessary to facilitate learning. Without the average how else would we start to study something that is as complex and diverse as the human body? It would be impossible. The average offers us a composite from which we can begin to explore, but in order to grow our knowledge base and create personal understanding and awareness, whether it be in medicine or yoga, we need to move beyond the average and into individual recognition and responsiveness.

This idea may seem contrary to what you have experienced in some yoga classes where the focus is on what we are calling the external, or top-down, approach. Group yoga classes often employ this approach out of necessity, offering a set of instructions based on the average in order to guide the class in an efficient way. Good yoga teachers are able to observe and evaluate whether or not the average instructions are working for the individual and then offer guidance to help a person adapt or modify the pose for her unique needs. This is often accomplished through refined verbal cues, the use of props, or hands-on assistance. When done skillfully, this approach allows for a variety of students with different body types to understand and employ strategies that work with their individual differences within a group class. The drawback to teaching to the average occurs when a teacher (or practitioner) adopts a belief that the average is something that is static, or believes it to be the end goal of practice, instead of a dynamic platform from which springs an endless variety of self-exploration and self-awareness.

Teaching the individual and teaching poses are fundamentally different. Instead of attempting to conform the body to an ideal shape (teaching poses), teachers can adapt the shape to support the individual body and the intentions of the person living in that body (teaching the individual). Taking this one step further, teachers can use the poses to help determine an individual's needs and serve as a guide for their practice. The ability to adapt the poses and be responsive to your individual goals is one of the primary learning outcomes desired for this book. We want you to grow into a practitioner empowered to create practices that support the activities of your life. We will do our best with the breath and pose variations offered in the coming sections to balance the need for clear instruction on the basics of a pose with the freedom for you to have your own experience. What we offer is a framework from which you can explore. Once you start exploring, the possibilities for awareness and related expressions of form are endless.

Some styles of yoga strictly dictate how to position the body in each pose. By now, you know us well enough to understand that we are less interested in a standardized definition of correct and are more interested in whether a pose is correct for you. This concept is especially important as you begin to sense and respond to your internal feedback loops and adapt yoga practices to suit your own intentions and needs.

As you use your yoga therapy practices to fine-tune your somatic sensibilities and be more responsive to the mind–body complex, you may start to encounter a variety of dormant, lingering characteristics. You might notice places where you can't let go of stress or tension, or you feel the physical or emotional remnants of old injuries, uncover unconscious holding patterns in the body and mind, unlock new ranges of motion, or discover previously unexamined aspects of your personality. Yoga therapy offers many opportunities to experience and explore your body and mind in new or forgotten ways.

When you come up against the feeling of "can't go any further" in a pose, you first have to ask yourself what "further" actually means to you. The modern world of postural yoga tends to place a high value on flexibility, which is neither practical nor necessary unless your intention for practice is to become a contortionist. This projected preference sometimes results in practitioners coveting or striving for a "yoga body," which our culture often projects to be lean and über bendy. Just as there is no ideal pose, there also is no ideal yoga body—just the perfectly imperfect body that you bring to the mat. We discourage you from coveting the body of another person. That body on the surface may appear more desirable, but you can never truly know what the cost–benefit ratio of living in that particular body actually is. It is far more beneficial to focus on being present in your own (and, in our opinion, rather amazing) body so that you can recognize and embrace your strengths while working skillfully to turn your challenges into compassionate learning opportunities.

Honoring Our Differences

At some point, no matter your experience or degree of practice, your asana might reach an end range. It may not be *the* end range, but something will prevent you from doing an asana like a photo, your teacher, or someone else in class. When that happens, it is beneficial to have context for the reasons behind it. In the yoga world, feeling stuck is often related to muscular tightness, but, of course, there may be more to it than what appears on the surface.

When the tissues around a joint are tight because of injury, previous conditioning, abuse, overuse, underuse, or misuse in daily life, you might feel tightness or tension in those areas. Although the interpretation of sensation can be subjective, the experience of muscular tightness in a pose is often described as a rubber band-like or feeling restricted. While it might be tempting to override the feedback of tight muscles and push through it to force a release or an opening, it can be counterproductive to do so. The tightness might be functional. For example, if you are a runner, strong calf and gluteal muscles propel you forward as you run. So while you might need to stretch them from time to time to prevent them from becoming too tight or weak (a tight muscle can also be a weak muscle), overstretching them could cause you to lose power when you run. Beyond that, forcing a tight muscle into a stretch can result in a tear or injury. From the perspective of a puzzle-solving nervous system, relaxing tight muscles can sometimes be a function of the nervous system figuring out how to do so. A muscle is more likely to relax when you feel safe. If you try to force an opening, the nervous system will likely say, "That's not safe," and tell the muscle to go into lockdown mode. For this reason, the concept of "less is more" often applies when your intention is to relax tight muscles in your practice. You are likely to engender openness and release when you pay attention, responding to your initial sensations and feedback loops.

The good thing about muscle tightness is that the body offers immediate feedback about what is too much. If you pay attention to the signals that your body gives rather than try to override them, you can work skillfully with your breath, slow down, back out, do a little less, and allow your nervous system to send the message that you are safe. If you are patient and allow that release to happen over time, some of those tight muscles that bother you might start to let go.

Joint structure may also keep you from going farther in a pose. The joints are crucibles of movement, and their structure will allow or prohibit certain movement patterns in the body. How the muscles and connective tissues pull on and shape the joint interface is important, but if those forces and inhibitions are removed through healthy stretching, corrective exercise, or manual manipulation, what remains are the bones and how their underlying structure allows or prohibits movement. While most of us possess the same joints in the same places, the subtle variations in angle of insertion or interface, space and length in the joint capsule, or size and shape of contacting surfaces can cause a wide variation in physical movement.

The crux of these considerations is that because everyone's skeleton is formed differently, no two people will ever have exactly the same pose shape or the same physical experience of a pose (figure 5.1). Attempting to do so, no matter the intention, may prove disheartening or even injurious, depending on the structure of the individual's joint. When you are unable to get into a certain variation of a yoga pose because of your bones, you can usually sense a "bony compression," meaning there is a hard stop and the joint refuses to go any farther. It also means that in order to go farther, other joints will have to move more to compensate. Pay attention to bony compression. When you get that hard stop, or stuck feeling, back off, look for your true range of motion, and then choose a variation accordingly.

Now that we have examined skeletal variety and its implications for yoga asanas, let's consider the muscles and fascia, which work with the bones and affect the physical experience of asanas. While your bony structures appear to be relatively inert (this is actually not the case from a molecular perspective), muscles, tendons, ligaments, and fascia are in a constant state of dynamism. With every movement you take, some parts are shortening and others lengthening—and the beauty of a regular, well-rounded yoga and movement practice is to ensure a balance between these two forces. From a larger perspective, achieving a balance between the two intrinsic capabilities of your muscles and fascia—strength and flexibility—is critical for overall wellness and healthy living. You don't want to be stronger than you are flexible or more flexible than you are strong. Flexibility without strength robs you of fine control and can exert unacceptable force or movement range on your joints, while strength without flexibility immobilizes the joints into particular patterns of movement at the loss of full range of motion.

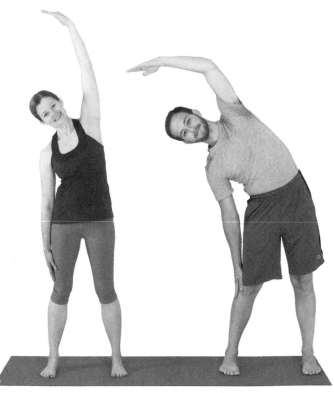

Figure 5.1 Both models have been practicing yoga for many years and are doing the standing side bend in a way that is appropriate for their underlying bone structures. The visual difference is remarkable.

Take, for example, the stereotype of a muscle-bound powerlifter. He may be able to bench- or shoulder-press hundreds of pounds, but as those muscles become so massive and powerful, how difficult it becomes to fit into a shirt! The term "muscle bound" can be quite literal. If muscles are trained only in a particular range or fashion, you can bind yourself to that movement at the loss of others.

Conversely, still sticking with stereotypes, picture a super flexible yoga practitioner who can put her feet behind her head and tie her arms in pretzels while performing twists. This makes for nice photographs, but what happens when those extremely open and flexible joints are made to bear weight? What happens when our fictitious yogi reaches for a heavy box high on a shelf? Muscles manipulate weight, but the bones bear it. Healthy bearing only happens if the joints are aligned functionally through the coordination and effort of the muscles and nervous system.

Skeletal variety is just one reason that one person's pose might need to be adapted or will look and feel very different from another's. Other reasons for variation and limitations exist. Use the following categories of awareness as a framework to assess why you might have difficultly executing certain movement patterns or yoga poses. Ultimately, we hope that you will use this information to more intelligently engage with the pose variations that we offer. When you are able to identify your individual challenges and work with them skillfully, you become empowered to create practices that are as dynamic, varied, interesting, and unique as you are.

Ligaments

Some body types have more or less collagen fibers. This means that a person can lean toward ligament laxity or ligament tightness. Where and how a person receives feedback about pose-related stretching or strengthening varies based on this sensory input. People leaning toward ligament laxity, or hypermobility, need to work on sensing where their body is in space and stopping themselves from going too far in pose. They might consider focusing less on stretching sensations and explore the strengthening variations of the poses outlined in upcoming chapters. People leaning toward tight ligaments, or hypomobility, might consider using the poses in the mobility or recovery sections. This is one example of how someone might adapt a yoga therapy practice to suit an individual physical need.

Soft-Tissue Approximation

This is a fancy way of saying that one part of the soft tissues of the body connects to another and stops the movement of a pose. One example might be people with larger buttocks and calf muscles. When they attempt to come back into child's pose, the buttocks hit the calf muscles and stop the backward movement, even though there might be more room in the joints or freedom in the muscles.

Previous Injuries

Scar tissue, adhesions, and bone fusions can impair the sliding surfaces between muscles and joints. This lack of movement often causes the affected person to perform a movement differently than the average person or to stop a movement before butting up against a restriction. For example, someone with a shoulder injury might have a difficult time raising his arms in a linear fashion up by his ears, but if he takes the arms out to the sides first and then up, he might be able to execute the movement.

Body Proportions

The combined proportions of a body can prohibit or enable someone to execute certain yoga poses. It is helpful to pay attention to how long or short your arms, torso, or legs are and the way that they may or may not come together when you attempt to perform certain yoga poses. When your proportions prohibit you from expressing a pose in a certain way, props like blocks, straps, and bolsters can be very helpful tools.

Fear and Psychology

Even though you might consider yourself healed from an old injury or emotional trauma, the imprint of it can remain in the body. For example, you might have the diagnosis of a slipped disc and remember the day when your back went into spasm as you bent over to pick something up. You associate that position of folding forward with the injury and avoid it because of the traumatic association. Yoga therapy can be an excellent tool to uncover these aspects of experience and work on them with skill and compassion.

Creating a Practice Based on Inquiry and Curiosity

The beautifully unique differences in our bodies make it difficult to write hard-and-fast sets of instructions for the poses in this book. We look to provide clear guidance and a framework from which you can begin to safely explore yoga asanas and then expand on them. Because of people's inherent differences, the mastery of cultivating individual awareness comes through time, inquiry, and understanding. You can ask yourself the following: *How* am I doing what I am doing? *Can* I do it differently? *What* does it feel like when I am doing it differently? Your differences can then become reference points for locating yourself so you can begin to understand how certain choices affect what you feel physically, energetically, mentally, or emotionally in yoga postures.

Through self-inquiry you open doors to limitless play and experimentation in your asana practice. The adaptations and pose experiences introduced in this work are limited only by the amount of space that we have to communicate. If we published every pose variation that we could envision, we would end up with more than a thousand pages—which wouldn't make for a very user-friendly experience! What we will offer are basic poses, movement experiences, and variations as they relate to creating five physical intentions for practice: **basic adaptations, mobility, strength, balance, and recovery.**

Your Practice Space

You can practice yoga anywhere. When you are designing an at-home practice, it is nice to have a quiet, clutter-free, well-ventilated space that can be converted or designated for yoga practice. If you live in a small space or find that parts of your space are cluttered and distracting, try covering them with a towel or sheet. You'll need enough space to put out your yoga mat and reach your arms out beyond your mat in all directions. Steer clear of sharp corners, and move valuable objects that you could accidentally fall into when doing balancing poses. Clear off a wall within your practice space so that you can easily explore wall variations. It is worth it to buy or borrow the props that we will use in this section. It is a small investment that will support your practice for a lifetime. When possible, we will offer household replacement options for certain props for a budget-conscious option.

If you don't already have one, it is worth it to purchase a yoga mat. Mats come in different thicknesses (1/8, 1/4, and 1/2 inch [3, 6, 12 mm]), weights, and densities. They are made of various materials (synthetics, rubber, jute, recycled materials) and come in different shapes. Most are rectangular, but there are circular options as well. The benefit of a thinner mat is it gives the feet firmer contact with the floor. This makes them useful for garnering feedback from the ground in standing and balancing poses. Thinner mats are also nice in carpeted practice spaces that are soft to begin with. The benefit of thicker mats is that they provide cushion for the joints, which can be nice when you are practicing on a hard surface. Rubber mats tend to have better grip, while some of the plastic options tend to be a little less tactile. Lots of options exist, so we suggest that you do research and pick a mat that is within your budget that also suits your personal and practice-space needs. From time to time, you may also want to experiment with practicing without a mat or on a variety of surfaces. You will use your body differently when you can't rely on the sticky quality of the mat to hold you in certain poses, or when you aren't restricted to practicing within the confines of the mat space.

Getting Started With Props

Yoga teachers and therapists often use props to create new learning outcomes for their students. Dedicated practitioners use them to support meaningful personal practices that evolve with their needs over the course of a lifetime. Different phases of life and their related intentions often require new strategies for practice, and having props to support those strategies opens up a variety of new possibilities. Here we will offer an overview of basic props that are available in most studios and gyms and their potential uses.

We tend to think of props as tools for learning, which means we look to use the right tool for the right job at the right time. The tool is only as good as the user's ability to apply it to the task at hand. And while the combinations are nearly infinite when you start to pair poses with all of the tools that we outline in this book, we will start by looking at six categories from which we can quantify the use of props before we apply them to the yoga asana explorations:

1. To support or create comfort and ease and release the body and mind.
2. To make a pose more accessible when you encounter a limit or restriction in the body.
3. To make a pose more accessible when you encounter a psychological or emotional limit or restriction.
4. To create positional joint awareness and refine postural alignments.
5. To solicit a specific kind of muscular awareness—activation or release—that will make a pose more or less muscularly challenging.
6. To facilitate breath and energy awareness.

Basic Props and Their Uses

In yoga therapy, props are used to create a variety of intentional experiences, facilitate individual awareness, and allow you to work skillfully with different body types and needs (figure 5.2). This means that you will need to engage with the props in an active way. We offer suggestions for intentions, along with interesting ways to explore them. But it is up to you to bring a sense of focus, curiosity, and play to the learning process. As you explore, please remember that the placement of a prop—even shifting just an inch or two (2.5-5 cm)—might appear subtle, but can have a large impact on your experience. It is important to have an open mind and to pay attention to your internal feedback mechanisms to help you discover or refine your personal intentions for exploration.

Wall

An ordinary wall is an excellent tool for training asana-related body awareness. It can guide muscular awakenings, help you to sense the skeleton, offer valuable proprioceptive feedback, create a platform from which to experience dynamic joint alignment, offer support when you are feeling unsteady in standing or balancing poses, and can be used for recovery and relaxation practices like legs against the wall (see chapter 6). While many traditional yoga poses use open-chain variations (figure 5.3a) to teach awareness of the extremities of the body along with muscular activity, the wall allows you to create closed-chain pose variations (figure 5.3b) that can awaken the core and allow you to better sense joint position. Do not assume that just because you are using the wall that the pose will become easier. It is correct to assume that the wall can be used to make a pose more accessible or

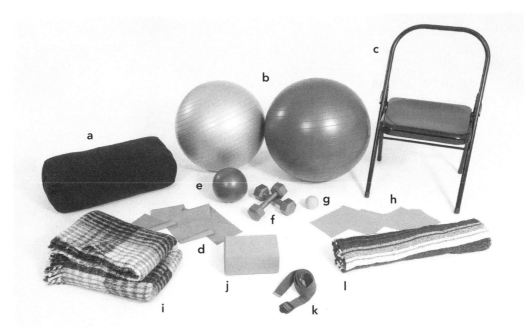

Figure 5.2 Basic props: (*a*) Rectangular bolster, (*b*) medium and large exercise balls, (*c*) backless yoga chair, (*d*) heavy resistance band, (*e*) small exercise ball, (*f*) light weights, (*g*) tennis ball, (*h*) light resistance band, (*i*) thick yoga blanket (Z-fold), (*j*) rubber block, (*k*) yoga strap, and (*l*) thin blanket (rolled).

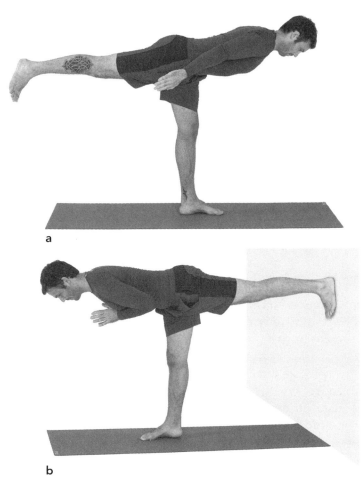

Figure 5.3 Warrior 3: In variation a, the back foot is disconnected from the wall (open chain) and the hands are apart at the sides of the body (open chain). In variation b, the back foot is plugged into the wall (closed chain) and the hands are pressed together in front of the body (closed chain).

create more ease in the body and mind, but it can also be used to create interesting and dynamic challenges.

Chair

Yoga poses can be adapted to be done in a seated position for people who have difficulty going from seated to standing or from the floor to upright. This approach, known as chair yoga, has helped make yoga poses available to a large portion of the population who might not otherwise have access. The chair can also be used as a balancing tool and offer support to a variety of postures outside of the chair-yoga realm.

Cushions

Types: Round or half-moon of different heights and densities
Household replacement: Pillows or sofa cushions
Typical uses: Cushions increase the height of a targeted region, alter the effect of gravity, and modify the relationship of the pelvis to other aspects of the pose.

Bolsters

Types: Cylinders or rectangles of different heights, lengths, and densities
Household replacement: Sofa cushions or folded blankets
Typical uses: Bolsters support the body in ways that facilitate relaxation, and they can adapt poses for a body that is restricted.

Blocks

Types: Rubber or cork, thick or thin, rectangular or oval
Household replacement: Thick, heavy books
Typical uses: Blocks can increase or decrease reach. They can also provide feedback for muscle activations in stabilizing poses, offer support for muscular release in recovery poses, help with balancing poses and creating asymmetrical pose variations, and create positional awareness.

Straps

Types: Buckle, clip, or metal ring; single strap; looped strap; various lengths
Household replacement: Necktie, scarf, or bathrobe belt
Typical uses: Straps extend reach, solicit muscular activity or awareness, support and guide movement, restrict movement, and create joint space.

Yoga Blankets

Types: Thin or thick; cotton, bamboo, wool, or made from recycled materials
Typical uses: Placed on top of a yoga mat, they protect joints from compression against the floor. Folded into round or rectangular shapes, they create support in poses when cushions or bolsters are unavailable, aren't the right fit, or don't quite meet needs. They can be used as a sliding mechanism for creative movement experiences and provide warmth in recovery or resting poses when body temperature drops.

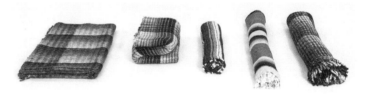

From left to right: Basic rectangle, zed, basic roll, paintbrush (thin blanket), and paintbrush (thicker blanket).

Blanket-Folding Basics

Basic rectangle: Fold one fringed end of your blanket to the other fringed end. Fold the fringe-to-fringe ends to meet again and create a rectangle.
Zed: Fold a basic rectangle into a Z-shape with three equal folds. This can double as a rectangular bolster when using a thick blanket.
Basic roll: Take a fringed end of the blanket and fold it in half two times to make a large rectangle. Starting with the fringed end, roll the blanket into a tight cylinder.
Paintbrush: Start with a blanket folded in a rectangle and roll it along the side perpendicular to the fringe so that it all lands at one end of a tight roll. This can double as a round bolster when using a thick blanket.

Resistance Bands

Types: Low, medium, or high resistance. Some have handles, others do not. The variations included in this book do not require handles.
Household replacement: None

Typical uses: Resistance bands create targeted muscular activity, introduce new options for strength training in the poses, and extend reach when a strap is not available.

Exercise Balls

Types: Small, medium, or large; weighted or unweighted
Household replacement: None
Typical uses: Exercise balls create an unstable platform from which to explore dynamic core awareness. Small balls are used to create targeted muscular activity, similar to the block. In some circumstances a ball can be used by itself or paired with a wall to provide a softer, more responsive, support mechanism. Larger exercise balls can be used as a light weight that can be held or passed overhead.

Weights

Types: Small and light (1-5 pounds [.5-2.5 kg])
Household replacement: Soup cans
Typical uses: Weights provide additional targeted strength training options for achieving maximal performance. There is no reason to replace strength training with yoga, but in some circumstances they can be integrated, as they are complementary disciplines.

One additional note: As much as we enjoy using props, there is something to be said for being able to do a personal practice without their assistance. It might be necessary to forego props if you are traveling or have limited access to equipment. We encourage you to explore variations of poses that employ props, along with those that do not.

Putting It All Together: Identification, Differentiation, and Integration in Mountain Pose

As you move into the next chapters, the yoga pose instructions will, by necessity, start to get more specific. Because you are likely to be motivated to practice in a group class, on your own, or in some combination of the two, you might at first find it challenging to identify what your movement inclinations and habits are. This is partially because you are processing the instructions that you are receiving, and the instructions will affect your actions and experiences in the movements. If you are a beginner, take time to first process the basic instructions. Once you develop familiarity with the basic instructions, you can start to identify how you interpret that particular instruction, becoming aware of patterns and themes that show up for you as you practice.

For example, you may notice that you tend initiate movement from the same place in your poses, feel restricted in other places, or avoid certain poses. It takes time, but this uncertainty is a fertile breeding ground from which awareness and empowered choices can eventually grow. At some point, you will be able to move from interpreting instruction to using the poses to learn more about who you are and how you move. Both beginner and experienced students experience advantages and challenges from this perspective. More experienced yoga practitioners often have already internalized a set of instructions or patterns for a pose. This means that the pose is familiar to them and they do it a certain way so the identification phase might be easier for them.

The differentiation phase could be more challenging for experienced practitioners, depending on their personality and mental flexibility and the beliefs about practice they have developed over the years. It's possible for beginners to have a more difficult time with the identification process but an easier time with the differentiation aspect because they are less set into a habit, belief, or expectation about their experiences of the poses and are therefore more receptive and yielding. Of course, these are just generalizations, and your experience of exploring options in practice might be different.

As you enter into the more pose-centric section of the book, we encourage you to continue with the intention of better understanding yourself. Inquiry is at the heart of what is possible in a yoga therapy practice. Regardless of where you are, know that the inquiry process that we are leading you through offers a safe framework from which you can explore. Be patient and kind to yourself as you practice. It will take some time for you to become aware of the movements you do subconsciously. Give yourself the time, space, attention, and rest that you need to develop this skill. As you take in more specific instructions for the basics of a pose and the variations that are offered, spend time getting a sense of how you are doing what we ask of you.

This next exploration will walk you through the process of identification, differentiation, and integration one more time as it relates to the mountain pose, adding the experience of a variety of targeted muscular activations and props into the mix. It will be from this expansive platform that we will start to focus a bit on more specific and detailed pose instructions.

EXPLORATION

Mountain Pose

This exercise is meant to highlight how you can apply the process of identification, differentiation, and integration into mountain pose with and without the use of props.

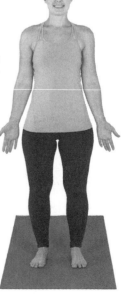

Identification Phase 1

In a standing position, close your eyes. Notice what you can sense about your posture from the inside out. The following are things to pay attention to:

- Feet. What parts of your feet are in more or less contact with the ground?
- Center of gravity. How are you finding balance?
- Muscular effort. What muscles are you using to hold yourself up?
- Tension. What parts of the body feel tight or stiff?

- Relaxation. What parts of the body feel soft or at ease?
- Emotional state. Are you happy, sad, frustrated, confident, confused, ashamed, overwhelmed, or excited in some way? What emotions are you feeling? How are those emotions reflected in your experience of your standing posture?
- Quality of mind. Is your mind busy or still? Agitated or lethargic? Sharp or dull? How many thoughts do you have and how quickly or slowly are they coming? How is your quality of mind reflected in your standing posture?
- Breath. How are you breathing while you are standing? How does your breath relate to the other areas that you have noticed?

Identification Phase 2

Now practice mountain pose. How does that differ from "just standing here"? Pay attention to all the same things you did in the previous exercise. How did they change when you gave the name mountain pose to what you were doing before (just standing here)?

Now that you have identified what the difference between "just standing here" and "mountain pose" means for you, move on to differentiating the physical intentions and experiences of mountain pose.

Differentiations Using Body Positions in Mountain Pose

Stance options: Try standing with your feet hip-width apart. What changes? Now try standing with your feet and legs together. What changes? Now try standing with your feet slightly wider than your shoulders. What changes?

Feet options: Place the weight of your body toward balls of your feet. Now try the heels. Press into the outer edges of the feet. Now try lifting the arches. Visualize a triangle on the bottom of the foot—the base is under the first and fifth toe; the point is in the center of the heel—and press equally into the points of the triangle. Grip the toes. Relax the toes. Pick the toes up and spread them out. What changes for you during each foot choice? Pay attention to the relationships between the feet, knees, and hips.

Hip-activity options: Bring the feet parallel, about hip's distance apart and firmly connect the triangle of both feet into the ground. Activate the legs by attempting to pull the feet towards each other without moving them, as if you were going to pull the mat together. The mat and the feet don't actually move, but you activate muscles with the action of pulling the legs towards each other. Now activate the legs by attempting to pull the feet away from each other without actually moving them, as if you were going to rip your mat apart. Now activate the legs by trying to turn your feet out like a duck without actually doing so, as if you were going to spiral the legs outward. Now attempt to turn your feet in toward your midline without actually doing so, as if you were going to spiral the legs inward. Attempt to pull your shins forward and thighs backward without moving the feet. Now attempt to pull your thighs backward and your shins forward without moving the feet. What changes for you during the different muscular activations? Pay attention to the changes in the relationships between the hips, knees, and feet.

Shoulder and arm options: Draw your shoulders back and down. Now let your shoulder blades spread apart. Place your arms by your sides in a relaxed fashion with your palms facing the sides of your legs. Imagine that you are sending your fingers down toward the earth. Press your palms into your legs. Now turn your palms forward. With the palms forward try the same options, pressing the fingers first down toward the ground and then the pinky fingers into the legs. Play with combining these activations and see what is interesting to you. Pay attention to the relationships between the arms, shoulders, spine, and core.

> continued

Differentiation Using Props in Mountain Pose

Wall: Bring your buttocks to the wall, keeping the feet under the hips. Press the back of your head lightly into the wall *(a)*. What changes? How does the rest of your body organize differently from this feedback? Now try different shoulder positions with the arms at the sides of the body and then press the arms back into the wall (palms away from the wall, palms toward the wall, palms toward each other) *(b)*. What changes with each shoulder position and the feedback of pressing the arms into the wall? Now do the same experiment with the arms reaching up by the ears.

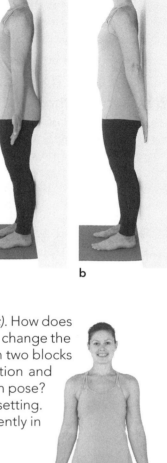

a   b

Block: Place a block between the thighs and gently squeeze it (*c*). How does that new feedback change your muscle awareness? How does it change the relationship between the feet, knees, and pelvis? Now stand on two blocks using the lower, flat setting. How does introducing this elevation and change of texture and feedback change your sense of mountain pose? Now place the block on top of your head—again on the low, flat setting. Can you keep it there or do you have to organize yourself differently in order to balance the block on top of the head?

c

Strap: With the feet hip-width apart, loop a yoga strap around the upper thighs. It can be snug but not so tight that it cuts into you (*d*). Press the outer edges of the thighs into the strap. How does that new feedback change your muscle awareness? How does it change the relationships between the feet, knees, and pelvis? Make a jacket by wrapping the strap at the midback under the shoulder blades. Pull the strap in front of you, leaving equal lengths on each side. Bring the front length of the straps over your shoulders and cross them behind you, creating an X on the back (*e*). Reach under and around to bring the straps back in front, giving them a gentle pull as you find the balance of support without restriction. When you find the appropriate tightness (again, it can be snug but not so tight that it cuts into you) buckle, loop, or tie the straps in the front of your body under the base of the sternum (*f*). How does this feedback change your experience of the pose?

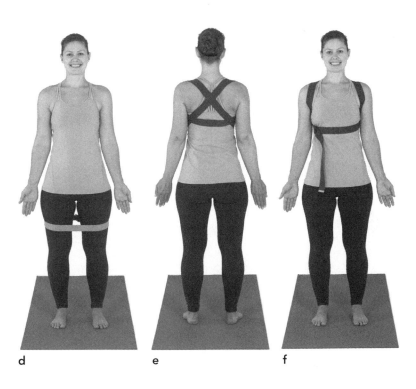

d   e   f

Integration

Come back into mountain pose without using any props. Think back on the feedback you received from the props while in mountain pose. Notice the impact introducing new muscle awareness and feedback has had on you. Revisit the points of observation from the identification phase of the exercise:

- Feet. What parts of your feet are in more or less contact with the ground?
- Center of gravity. How do you find balance?
- Muscular effort. What muscles are you using to hold yourself up?
- Tension. What parts of the body feel tight or stiff?
- Relaxation. What parts of the body feel soft or at ease?
- Emotional state. How is your emotional state reflected in your experience of your standing posture?
- Quality of mind. How is that reflected in your standing posture?
- Breath. How do you breathe while you are standing? How does your breath relate to the other areas that you have noticed?

What new awareness have you gained from using the body and prop modifications to help you stand with more interest, integrity, or ease? How can the awareness translate into daily life and the activities that you love?

It might seem like you just spent a lot of time on one pose, but our hope is that the exercise gives you a better sense of what your options are when standing in mountain pose. Of course, the differentiations that we offer here are not exhaustive. Given the chance, we could probably write a whole book just on mountain pose! While it's not always the most obvious or flashiest thing to do, it is important to remain open to revisiting the basics from time to time. The habits that you have in everyday activities such as breathing, sitting, standing, walking, and sleeping are a breeding ground for improved awareness that can carry over into your movement practices and vice-versa. Being able to mark and understand those things is the start of being empowered to embody new options and effect positive changes when it is helpful or needed.

If it has not been emphasized enough, we'll say it again here: This book contains many considerations and instructions for pose experiences, but it is certainly not the end-all of these experiences. After some time, you will begin to notice specific habits that you have in different poses. If you pay attention, you may also notice that those same habits play themselves out in other activities in your life. Our greatest hope is that we inspire you to *identify* how your movement habits reveal themselves, *differentiate* your movement patterns through inquiry and variety, *integrate* what you learn, and then continue to apply what you have learned to enhance your experience of life's activities.

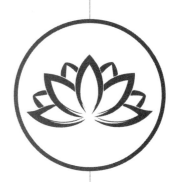

six
Breathing and Relaxation

As mentioned in chapter 4, breath is central to who we are. It relates to all of the activities of our lives. Our ability to work, think, sleep, exercise, or interact with others is in some way dependent on our breath. One could argue that breathing is the core pattern of our lives that drives all other patterns. Breathing is one of those things that we do automatically; we often don't think about it until something goes wrong.

That lack of consciousness can result in being stuck in breathing patterns that are at best unhelpful and at worst dysfunctional, creating problems for us in life. Maybe you are stuck in a breathing pattern that causes anxiety. Maybe your breathing pattern does not allow you to adapt to different situations, relates to addictive behaviors, or leaves you feeling depleted. Maybe your pattern detracts from, rather than enhances, your experience of favorite activities. These are just some of the reasons that you might chose to consciously engage with the breath. Because breathing can be voluntary or automatic, the breath is an aspect of your physiological experience that you can bring into your conscious awareness.

Breathing and Yoga

Breathing is also central to yoga therapy practices. You might remember that we mentioned earlier one of the branches of the eightfold path of yoga called pranayama, which is often translated as "breath control" or "breath mastery." While it might be appealing to think of controlling the breath, another way to consider it from a yoga therapy perspective is attempting to remove the obstacles between you and a free, adaptable breath. To free your breath, you first need to identify your current breathing patterns. Hopefully you have already begun this process through the positional breath exploration in chapter 4. If you haven't already been playing with positional breath awareness, now might be a good time to revisit that exploration.

The next step is to become more aware of your breathing patterns in daily life. Spend time simply observing your breath. Observe it when you are relaxed, at work, with your family, stressed, close to someone you love, and when you are close to someone you don't like. Can you observe your breath during all of those interactions?

Do you notice when your breathing changes as you go from one context to the next? Does your breathing change before you get stressed, or do you get stressed and then your breath changes? These and many other observations give you a chance to play with new patterns.

Wouldn't it be great if you acquired different breathing patterns to match different situations? Imagine adapting your breath when you are at work, with your family, stressed, exercising, playing, or with people you don't like. You may be thinking, "Yes, I want to change! How do I do more than just notice my breathing pattern?" The answer is to use this awareness to create the change itself.

Once you are aware of your breathing patterns, you can start playing with your breath. Notice the word *playing*. Often in yoga and other methods of breath work, the focus tends to be on control. For example, we are told to breathe in for so many seconds, hold, breathe out for so many seconds, hold. Breathe in when you do this, and breathe out when you do that. All those instructions are well meant, but sometimes they cause unnecessary worry and tension, especially in people who are already suffering from information overload. When you try to control your breath, you run the risk of layering a stressful, dysfunctional, or ineffective pattern onto the pattern that is already there. Instead, let's deconstruct and play with breathing patterns in various combinations.

Play also implies options for variety. The freedom to choose is a joyful activity for the development of the nervous system. This variety is also required of the breath if you are to navigate different life situations and experiences. Trust that after the playtime, the nervous system will begin to choose the pattern that is the most efficient for a particular circumstance. The better you can adapt your breath to different yoga pose experiences, the better you will be able to function in *all kinds* of life and movement situations. After all, it may not be beneficial to breathe the same way when your boss yells at you as when you hug your spouse, or to breathe the same way when you are playing tennis as when you are running! Differentiating breathing patterns gives the nervous system options so that you can respond to the situation at hand effectively. By playing with variety, you gather new possibilities for the breath as it relates to your life activities and experiences.

This next section offers you breath-play practices to get you started. Remember that play implies you don't do things in the same way over and over. Your nervous system does not like too much repetition and will not become adaptable if you replicate an experience without variety. Play also indicates a relaxed sense of awareness. See whether you can explore the exercises without creating strain or tension in the body. Use the following options as starting points, and then experiment with new breathing variations as they become more accessible and available to you.

It will be more meaningful for you to explore the breathing differentiations that follow if you have a baseline understanding of your current patterns. This will allow you to make comparisons in order to see what is changing. It will also offer a better understanding of how you can integrate the new breathing options into your favorite life activities.

Once you have identified your baseline, you can use that awareness in exploratory practice. The following intentions for breath can be explored in reclined, belly-down, kneeling, seated, or standing positions. Each change of position will provide new potential for awareness and adaptability.

Baseline Breath

1 Observe your natural rhythm of breath without attempting to change it. What is the location of the breath? Where do you feel it in your body? Front or back? At the side? Down low? Up high?

2 What is the quality of the breath? Rapid or slow? Shallow or deep? Complete or incomplete?

3 Is there an emotion or feeling associated with the breath?

4 Do you have a visual impression or image that goes with the breath?

5 What is the phrasing of the breath? What is the length of the inhalation vs. the exhalation? The length of the pauses between them?

Mouth and Nose Breath

With just the intention of slowing your inhalations and exhalations, explore the following options to see whether you can determine what your habit is. Also notice how the options affect your physical well-being, emotional state, energy level, quality of mind, and spiritual sense of self.

1 Breathe in through the nose, out through the mouth.

2 Breathe in through the mouth, out through the nose.

3 Breathe in through the nose, out through the nose.

4 Breathe in through the mouth, out through the mouth.

Inhalation and Exhalation

1 Try to make your inhalation longer than your exhalation. Play with different counts.

2 Try to make your exhalation longer than your inhalation. Play with different counts.

3 Try to make your inhalation and exhalation about the same length.

4 Bring your attention to a sense of fullness on the inhalation. Try to do this without creating strain or tension in the body. Keep the intention settled on fullness for the inhalation and allow the exhalation to happen however it happens.

5 Bring awareness to a sense of emptying the lungs on the exhalation. Keep the intention on a complete exhalation. (You might be surprised how much there is to release.) Allow the inhalation to happen however it happens.

6 Bring a relaxed sense of fullness and completeness to both the inhalation and exhalation. Allow the awareness to land on the pauses that happen between them.

Breath Location

1 Try to allow the breath to inflate the front of the torso on the inhalation and deflate the front of the torso on the exhalation.

2 Try to allow the breath to inflate the back of the torso on the inhalation and deflate the back of the torso on the exhalation.

> continued

3 Try to allow the breath to move sideways into the torso on the inhalation and deflate the sides of the torso on the exhalation.

4 Try to sense in your skull the subtle expansion of the inhalation and contraction of the exhalation.

5 Keeping the relaxed sense of fullness of inhalation and exhalation, see whether you can sense the gentle opening of the pelvic floor that happens during the inhalation and closing of the pelvic floor that happens during each exhalation.

6 Experiment with breathing into the abdomen and low back, allowing them to inflate with the inhalation and deflate with the exhalation.

7 See whether you can breathe into the rib cage, allowing it to expand front, back, and sideways during the inhalation and deflate during the exhalation.

8 Try three-dimensional breathing, allowing the breath to inflate the front, back, and sides of the torso on the inhalation and deflate the same areas on the exhalation.

EXPLORATION
Three-Part Breathing

The following are three variations of the yogic three-part breath. As you explore, think of an intentionally slow and gradual buildup of the inhalation, along with a slow and gentle release of the exhalation.

Part 1: Top to Bottom and Bottom to Top

1 Try to take a smooth inhalation that links the following areas from bottom to top in this order: abdomen, rib cage, upper chest. Release the air slowly and smoothly in this order: upper chest, rib cage, abdomen.

2 Try to take a smooth inhalation that links the following areas from top to bottom in this order: upper chest, rib cage, abdomen. Release the air slowly and smoothly in this order: abdomen, rib cage, upper chest.

Part 2: Three-Part Breath With Retention

1 Using the version of the three-part breath (steps 1 or 2) that you find the most interesting, allow a 3- to 5-second pause between the inhalations and the exhalations.

2 Using the version of the three-part breath that you find the most interesting, hold the breath in the body at the top of the inhalation. You can determine the length of time that you want to retain the breath. Pay attention to the feelings and reactions caused by holding the breath in. Use your ability to stay sensitive to your reactions, mentally present, and physically relaxed as markers for how long is appropriate for you.

3 Using the version of the three-part breath that you find the most interesting, hold the breath out of the body at the bottom of the exhalation. You can determine the length of time that you want to hold the breath out. Pay attention to the feelings and reactions caused by holding the breath out. Use your ability to stay sensitive to your reactions, mentally present, and physically relaxed as markers for how long is appropriate for you.

Part 3: Three-Part Breath With Alternating Nostrils

1 Using the version of the three-part breath that you find most interesting, try breathing into the right nostril and out of the left, using your thumb to gently close off each nostril as you go. Once you have a sense of it, try reversing the pattern by breathing into the left nostril and out of the right.

Integrating Breath Awareness Into Daily Life

As you become more familiar and mindful of your breath, you can use it as a barometer of sorts, a way to check in with yourself to see how you are doing. This is a way to become more present and mindful of the breath in a natural state, without imposing patterns or ideas of right or wrong onto it. Note that the simple act of intermittent observation changes your experience of the breath. Check in as often as you can to become aware of how you are breathing in different life situations. See whether you can cultivate a sense of curiosity along with an attitude of compassion toward yourself while doing this. Look for breath patterns to see how they reflect your life experience. The following are times you could check in:

- Upon waking and transitioning into the day
- Driving to or from work
- During the more mundane daily chores
- Before, during, and after meals
- During happy situations (e.g., a deal at work went through, hearing good news from a friend, hearing a favorite song on the radio)
- During challenging situations (e.g., while stuck in traffic, during a confrontation with a family member, when the dishwasher breaks)
- Before, during, and after movement practices
- Preparing for bed and sleep

Breathing in Yoga Poses

A variety of opinions on what "correct" or "yogic" breathing is exists among both ancient and modern yoga traditions. This leads to conflicting information on if, when, where, why, and how you should or should not breathe during yoga poses. We have theories as to why this might be, but we will focus here on what we have been teaching over the years: Just as there is no one correct way to breathe in life (and we hope that the explorations so far have illuminated this for you), there is also no one correct way to breathe in a yoga pose.

There is only what is correct in the moment that the person experiences her breath relationship with all of her physical, emotional, energetic, mental, and spiritual realities. Yes, some ways of breathing might better support a particular movement pattern—for example, inhaling into a backbend or exhaling into a forward bend—but from our perspective of the nervous system figuring out movement puzzles, pairing different patterns of breath with your yoga poses is just as important. It is as interesting and worthwhile to exhale as you enter a given yoga pose as it is to inhale into that same pose. Once you have spent time identifying what your existing breathing habits are and have familiarized yourself with the differentiations, you will be able to decide for yourself how and when different breathing strategies may be useful in your yoga pose practice. Of course, the freedom of choice that comes with breath awareness will integrate into the other activities of your life.

Breath Intentions in Child's Pose

1 Come into your preferred version of child's pose for 1 to 2 minutes (*a*). Observe your breath in its natural state without changing it or superimposing a specific pattern or intention onto it. What is your tendency for breathing here? Where do you feel the breath more or less? Where does your breath feel restricted vs. free? How does your breath reflect your emotional state? How does your breath reflect your current state of mind? Make a note of what you noticed.

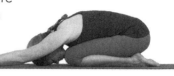

a

- While in your preferred version of child's pose, try the following breathing strategies. See how they affect your physical, emotional, or mental experience in the pose.
- Breathe with the intention of filling the entire back of your body with breath. The breath raises the back of the body skyward during the inhalation and lowers it earthward during the exhalation.
- Breathe with the intention of filling up the sides of the body with breath. Allow the breath to expand the sides of the body away from the spine during the inhalation and toward the spine during the exhalation.
- Breathe with the intention of inflating the area around the abdomen and low back, inflating with the inhalation and deflating with the exhalation.
- Breathe with the intention of filling the entire torso—front, back, and sides. Try inhaling from top to bottom and exhaling from bottom to top.
- Breathe with the intention of filling the entire torso—front, back and sides. Try inhaling from bottom to top and exhaling from top to bottom.

Now try these variations of child's pose partnered with breathing explorations.

2 Knees together, rounded child's pose, arms by side (*b*): Breathe with the intention of filling the entire back of your body with breath. The breath raises the back of the body skyward during the inhalation and lowers it earthward during the exhalation.

3 Side-bend child's pose (*c*): Breathe with the intention of filling the sides of the body with breath. Allow the breath to expand the sides of the body away from the spine during the inhalation and toward the spine during the exhalation.

4 Wide-knee child's pose, relaxed arms by ears: Breathe with the intention of inflating the area around the abdomen and low back, swelling that area during the inhalation and lowering it during the exhalation.

5 Active reaching child's pose (*d*): Breathe with the intention of expanding the rib cage forward, backward, and sideways in the inhalation and drawing it back toward the spine in the exhalation.

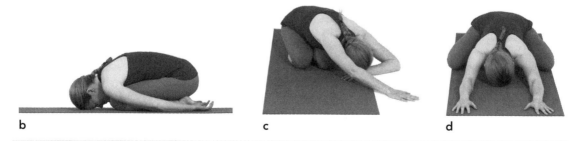

b   c   d

Did you notice that when you changed your intention for breath, your experience of other aspects (physical, emotional, energetic, mental, spiritual) of the pose changed too? How about when you changed your position with the breath? We encourage you to explore the yoga pose variations offered in the next chapters in tandem with your developing breath knowledge so that you can observe, adapt, and be responsive to your breath instead of continually superimposing the same pattern, attempting to control your breathing, or breathing "correctly." Instead, think of breath options and notice how they can affect your experience of a given pose. Inquire into your breath in moments of stillness and movement with a sense of compassion, wonder, freedom, and receptivity. Trust in the intelligence of your body and its capacity for self-healing. Whenever you are finished exploring, come back to the breath observation that you started with and notice what you have learned.

Because you can breathe in so many ways, pairing breath with movement and yoga poses creates the potential for nearly infinite combinations of gross to subtle experiences in your practice. As you progress into your personal yoga therapy practice, we encourage you to explore the possibilities of your breath so that in time you can consciously choose meaningful, helpful breath-centered experiences for all the activities of your life.

Relaxation and Meditation

At this point in your explorations, you have probably noticed that certain breathing patterns are more or less helpful in guiding you toward a relaxed feeling in the body or a clear state of mind. As you explore the connection between breathing and relaxation, it is important to recognize that whether or not a breathing pattern helps you to relax depends on context. For example, if you are in a completely relaxed state, simply observing the natural rhythm of your breath, attempting to do deep breathing might shift you into a state of alertness. Conversely, if you have been doing a lot of physical activity or are experiencing anxiety, a slower, deeper breath could help you to relax, lower your heart rate, or better manage your emotions. That being said, exploring a slower, deeper breath is often the gateway to exploring the practices of relaxation and meditation.

To the outside observer, the practices of relaxation and meditation might look fairly simple. It appears as if everyone is either sitting quietly doing nothing (meditation) or taking a nap (relaxation). Yet anyone who has tried to do either can tell you that it is far more complex than it appears on the surface. Many will also tell you that they have found both practices to be excellent antidotes for what happens to the body, mind, and spirit as a result of living in an overstimulated, fast-paced, multitasking world. If you want to further integrate what you have learned about the many layers of yourself from the yoga therapy explorations, both are essential tools that will support you in that intention.

What is the difference between relaxation and meditation? The simplest way to differentiate the two is to say that relaxation focuses more on the body, while meditation focuses more on the mind. It is helpful to think about breathing, relaxation, and meditation as a continuum of practices. Deep breathing starts the process of relaxation, and in turn relaxation facilitates the process of quieting the mind. Quieting the mind leads to compassionate self-awareness and the ability to witness and observe your thoughts and feelings without having to judge or act on them.

This can lead to a state of tranquility, where thoughts and feelings drop away. The ensuing silence and stillness become the meditative state.

This continuum of practices results in a paradoxical state of alert awareness and complete relaxation in which you can shift from thinking and doing to feeling and being. In this space, brainwaves shift and the nervous system downregulates. Here you have a tremendous opportunity for physical, emotional, mental, and spiritual healing. Symptoms of stress diminish, the immune system gets a boost, blood pressure lowers, blood flow increases, muscular tension decreases, concentration and mood improve, and fatigue is lowered. When you stop to think about it, it is really quite amazing to think how little physical effort these practices require in comparison to the many benefits that they offer.

Just as there is no one correct way to do a yoga pose, there also is no one correct way to meditate. Techniques for meditation tend to fall into six categories: breath, visualization, mantra, prayer, mindfulness, and contemplative inquiry. We will focus on a breath meditation in the following exploration, but if you want to determine which style of meditation works best for you, we highly recommend that you read *Meditation for Your Life: Creating a Plan That Suits Your Style* by Robert Butera, PhD (Bob is our YogaLife Institute colleague and Kristen's husband). One of his areas of specialization is guiding people to uncover their personal meditation style. As the Director of the Comprehensive Yoga Therapy program in which we both teach, his approach to teaching meditation fits very well with the concepts that we have explored in this book.

Strategies for relaxation can also vary. In the following exploration, we use a combination of breath, visualization, and mindfulness to help you facilitate a relaxation response. Other techniques include body scanning (focusing on different points in the body), progressive muscle relaxation (purposely contracting and relaxing muscles), autogenics (a form of self-hypnosis), affirmation (internally repeating a positive mantra), sound relaxation (listening to recorded music, singing bowls, or other soothing sounds), and guided imagery (someone guides the practitioner on a visual journey). All of these approaches are worth exploring in order to discover a style of relaxation that it is effective and works well for your disposition and needs.

If you are new to relaxation or meditation, it might seem challenging at first. But many new practitioners pick up the benefits very quickly. Students often experience profound and immediate changes in themselves as a result of consistently cultivating these practices. If this is your first time trying them, remember that it is a process that some people master faster and easier than others. If your disposition leans toward firing on all cylinders all the time, it might take a while to develop the skill of conscious relaxation or to find a meditation technique that works for you. Take it in increments and give the practices time and space to unfold for you organically.

Remember that you can practice relaxation and meditation alone or as part of a well-rounded yoga therapy practice. Many people find that the ability to slow down comes through doing some kind of yoga asana or movement practice before attempting to relax or meditate. Play around with trying the practices at different times to see when you are more receptive to it. If you find yourself unable to truly relax or meditate, remember that the simple act of lying down and focusing on the natural rhythm of your heartbeat or breath will allow you to slow down and observe different aspects of your body, mind, and spirit with less reactivity. As always, be patient and kind with yourself as you explore.

TIP: An eye pillow or small rolled towel covering the eyes reduces unnecessary stimulation during relaxation.

Reclined: Come into a fully reclined position. If needed for comfort, place a small blanket or pillow under the knees and a blanket roll under the neck. Focus on an unforced, slow, and relaxed rhythm of abdominal breath. Hands can rest at the sides of the body on floor with the palms up or on the body (as pictured).

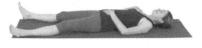

Belly down: In a belly-down position, place the arms bent at the top of the mat with forehead resting on stacked hands. Hips and feet can stay together behind the body or come out wider toward the outer edges of the mat.

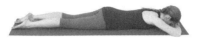

Side lying: Lie on your side. Bend the top knee and prop the shin on a bolster or blanket stack. Use a blanket roll, block, or pillow under the head if needed.

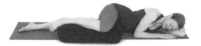

Legs on blocks and bolster: Place three blocks on their medium (long and narrow) setting lengthwise at one end of the mat. Set the bolster on top of the blocks. From a reclined position, place the backs of the lower legs onto the bolster and allow them to relax into the support.

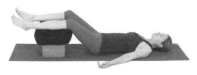

Legs on a chair: Drape a chair with a folded blanket. From a lying position on the floor, place the backs of the lower legs onto the seat of the chair. If you are practicing at home, you can practice this variation with a sofa as well.

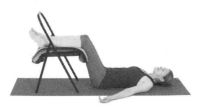

Legs on a ball: From a reclined position, bend both knees and drape the backs of the lower legs over a medium or large exercise ball. Draw the ball up towards the buttocks, allowing the backs of the thighs to also be supported by the ball.

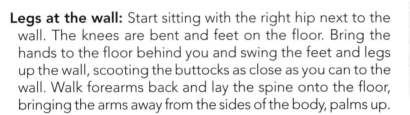

Legs at the wall: Start sitting with the right hip next to the wall. The knees are bent and feet on the floor. Bring the hands to the floor behind you and swing the feet and legs up the wall, scooting the buttocks as close as you can to the wall. Walk forearms back and lay the spine onto the floor, bringing the arms away from the sides of the body, palms up.

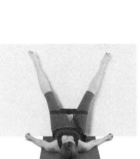

Legs at the wall, strapped variation: Loop a strap around the outer edges of both legs at the thigh or shin level. Make the strap narrow and firm enough that the legs are able to relax into the feedback and support.

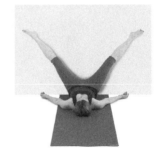

Legs at the wall, wide variation: Open the legs out in a V-shape.

Legs at the wall, bolster or block variation: Place a bolster or block lengthwise under the pelvis.

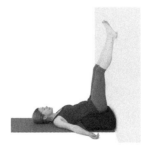

TIP: Just as there is no one right way to do a yoga pose, there also is no one singular way to sit for meditation. It often requires finesse for practitioners to find a position that allows the spine to stay upright without being rigid. Look for a variation that allows the spine (with a natural lumbar curve), shoulders, head, and neck to stack directly over the pelvis. The position for the lower half of the body should feel steady, stable, and, most important, sustainable while sitting for an extended period of time. Back, shoulder or neck pain, loss of sensation in the legs, and pins and needles in the feet are all indicators that you may need to explore alternative positions.

Simple crossed leg: Start seated with the legs straight in front of you. Bend the right knee and bring the right foot toward the left buttock. Do the same with the left leg, bringing it in front of the right. Keep the head, neck, spine, and pelvis stacked as you sit. Hands can rest on the thighs with the palms up or down.

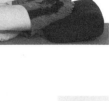

On a block, blanket, or pillow: Place a folded blanket, horizontal yoga block, or meditation cushion behind you. Sit on the edge of the prop to help angle the front of the pelvis toward the floor and find an appropriate lumbar curve.

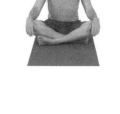

At the wall: Sit with the back of the body against a wall for feedback and support. You can also try a large exercise ball, bolster, or block at the wall behind you for different types of feedback or support in specific areas.

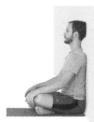

Chair: Start seated near the front edge of a chair, feet on the floor or on blocks. Tuck a bolster behind the torso for support if needed. Sit on the edge of the chair to help angle the front of the pelvis toward the floor and find an appropriate lumbar curve.

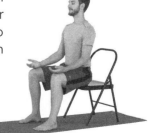

Kneeling: Start in a table position with the knees together and a small blanket roll underneath the front of the ankles with tops of the feet on the floor. Sit the buttocks back to the heels. The spine stays upright in active neutral.

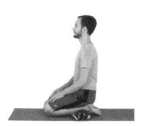

Kneeling, propped: Straddle a bolster, blanket roll, or blanket roll stacked on top of a bolster.

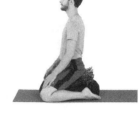

Kneeling with a blanket behind the knees: Place a large blanket roll or bolster behind the knees to help create a little extra joint space.

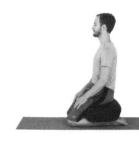

Heel to heel: Bring the right heel in towards the groin. Place the heel of the left foot in front of the right. At some point during meditation, switch which leg is in front.

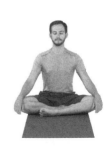

Half lotus: From the simple crossed-leg position, draw the right foot into the left thigh crease and move the left foot toward the right buttock. At some point during the meditation, switch which leg is on top.

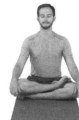
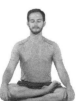

Breathing, Relaxation, and Meditation

1 Start in a comfortable reclined position, using any props that you need to support your body and facilitate the ability to rest. If you cannot find a comfortable reclined position for relaxation, feel free to explore other options such as belly down or side lying.

2 Set an intention for your relaxation and meditation practice. If you are struggling to find an intention, try concepts such as integration, rejuvenation, peacefulness, freedom, surrender, trust, faith, clarity, or simply paying attention to your natural breathing rhythm.

3 Close your eyes. Bring your awareness to the back of the body and the weight of it against the floor. Let the body be held by the earth, and trust in the support that it offers. If you find parts of the body that are unable to relax, surround that area with a healing light or color. If visualization doesn't work, try using intentional exhalations to try to soften or let go of holding in those areas.

4 Notice where in your body your attention lands. Try shifting your attention to your breath, slowing as it comes in through the nose and out through the nose. Keep the mouth closed and the jaw soft. Visualize breathing in 3D into the areas in and around the abdomen and low back; allow the breath to move forward, backward, and sideways in those areas. Keep the breath relaxed and easy, with the exhalations slightly longer than the inhalations. Explore this style of breathing for a few minutes. If you find that your attention wanders, gently bring it back to the breath.

5 Shift your awareness to your thoughts and emotions, paying attention to the obvious things that you might be feeling. Can you observe your thoughts and emotions without judgment or reaction? If you are coming up against a specific obstacle, visualize the obstacle leaving you during your exhalation, and bring in new possibilities or a positive opposite quality during your inhalation. If you get hung up on a particular thought or series of thoughts, visualize them as passing clouds being moved out of your mental sphere by a gentle breeze. Stay in this observational space for as long as it is helpful. If observing your thoughts and emotions proves to be too difficult or not relaxing, come back to your natural breathing rhythm. Watch your body breathe or simply do nothing. Rest.

6 Stay in relaxation from 5 to 15 minutes.

7 When you are ready to shift out of relaxation, do it slowly using gentle, deep breaths. Connect the deeper breaths with small movements in the hands and feet, and explore movements that come naturally to help you transition from resting to waking consciousness.

8 Roll over to one side and stay there for a minute or two, continuing to breathe as you give the body and mind a little time to transition from relaxation into being upright. As you come upright you can shift into a meditation practice. If you do not plan to meditate, try to keep a relaxed attitude during the transition.

9 Come upright into a comfortable meditative seat. Shift your awareness back to the breath. Observe your breath in its natural state, without changing it or superimposing a specific pattern or intention upon it. Notice the subtle rise and fall of the breath in the body. Feel the subtle warmth of the inhalations and the coolness of the exhalations passing over the top of the lip. If you are disturbed by thoughts or emotions, notice the disturbance and return to observing the breath. Eventually, you may not need to use the breath as an anchor to stay present and find yourself in a pure meditative state.

10 Sit in meditation from 5 to 20 minutes.

Breathing, relaxation, and meditation practices are paramount to living a fully integrated life. They might not seem as compelling as the yoga poses themselves, but they are an essential part of the complete yoga experience. Without them, yoga poses are just exercises. With them, you connect the ability to breathe, relax, and harness the power of the mind in a variety of intentions in yoga poses; you embody a practice that has the power to transform you physically, emotionally, mentally, and spiritually. We will continue exploring the transformational potential of yoga therapy practices in chapters 8, 9, and 10, but before that happens, we will shift the dialogue to injury prevention from two perspectives. First we will examine how to avoid injuring yourself in yoga poses, and then we will explore how to use your yoga therapy practices to prevent injuries in other aspects of your life. With that additional information, you will be well prepared to make exciting new connections among your body, mind, and spirit.

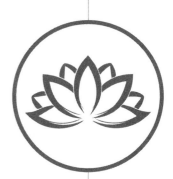

seven
Preventing Injury

The Man Who Broke His Thigh Bone Doing Yoga: 'Severe injury is only normally seen in car crash victims,' doctors say.

This was a headline in the *Daily Mail* (a British newspaper). The person was doing a complex posture and fractured his femur. Many people reading this would assume that yoga is not safe. Big news! People love the big headlines, and this article was based on a peer-reviewed article in the *British Medical Journal Case Reports*. But how many people looked at the original article to get the facts? Well, we did.

The journal article mentions that this person had previous microfractures of his femur and osteopenia, considered to be a precursor to osteoporosis. So the person in the article had a weakened bone condition and had hurt himself previously but continued to do advanced postures. When reporting on yoga injuries, as with many topics, newspapers are often more interested in a sensational headline than an in-depth investigation of what happened and why. That said, injuries do happen during yoga asana practice.

Yoga is safe, but practitioners do get hurt from time to time. The *BMJ Case Reports* article states that the authors could identify only three published studies that reported fractures occurring during yoga and that "while yoga injuries are not that uncommon, the most common adverse events are musculoskeletal related, mainly minor ligament or muscle injuries that recover fully without intervention" (Moriarity, Ellanti, and Hogan 2015).

Most yoga injuries are indeed minor, but occasionally significant injuries occur. And lately those injuries have been getting as much press coverage as the health benefits millions of people enjoy from yoga. People also need to remember that when they read about yoga injuries, the reports are talking about what happens during asana practice, which is a small part of a comprehensive yoga therapy approach.

So why do injuries happen in yoga? There are lots of theories, but not many clear answers. Theories have suggested people pushing themselves too hard, teachers who are not well educated, and people having preexisting conditions that flare up during yoga. A study by Fishman, Saltonstall, and Genis (2009) tried to answer this question. They sent out a questionnaire to yoga teachers and yoga therapists in several countries and received 1,336 responses. The first question was "Please estimate what you believe to be the percentage of people who do yoga (primarily) for each of the following reasons."

The number one reason for practicing yoga was fitness and general health (53.4 percent), followed by peacefulness, liberation, and enlightenment (18.2 percent). However, reason number three was a remedy for specific medical solutions (16 percent), and number four was a remedy for emotional problems (9.7 percent). Thus, 16 percent of students might be doing yoga for solutions to medical problems, and nearly 10 percent might be stressed and therefore at an increased risk of injury. Considering those numbers and the fact that yoga has been touted as a remedy for osteoporosis, stress, back pain, neck pain, and countless other ailments, maybe we should change the question from "Why do people get injured in yoga?" to "Why don't more people get injured in yoga?"

The next survey question asked whether there are more injuries among yoga practitioners today than in the past. Thirty-nine percent of those surveyed answered yes. The following are the top reasons:

- Excessive student effort (81.4 percent)
- Inadequate teacher training (68.2 percent)
- More people doing yoga overall (65.4 percent)
- Unknown preexisting conditions (59.5 percent)
- Larger classes (47 percent)

Of course, we should be concerned about all yoga injuries, but for this book, we will mainly concern ourselves with the excessive student effort and unknown preexisting medical conditions.

To be more aware of your body, you can go back to the concepts of **identification**, **differentiation**, and **integration**. By identifying what you are doing when you assume an asana, you have already started becoming more aware. By becoming more aware, you can become more mindful of the effort you are using—overall endeavor as well as where in the body you can sense the strain. The places where you sense excessive effort could be the areas of the body where you are at increased risk for injuries. After identifying areas of excessive effort, you can then differentiate in the asana to become aware of how you can modify it to lessen the strain. When you decrease the excessive effort, you will be able to safely continue and modify your asana practice throughout life.

As mentioned in chapter 5, we are all different. We have different habits, skeletal structures, and connective tissue extensibility. Trying to make our body fit the pose instead of making the pose fit the body can lead to injuries. When the person next to us can do the pose easily, can hold the pose longer, or is more flexible than us, we often become competitive. As a matter of fact, when the yoga instructor survey asked about what factors might cause an injury, the number one response was ego and number two was excessive effort. Also high on the list was inadequate instructions, pressure from the teacher or group, and undisclosed prior conditions. So if we drop our egos, receive adequate instructions, and disclose prior medical conditions, then injuries should decline. You as a student can affect all these factors.

Take Charge of Your Health and Safety

When you walk into a yoga class where the teacher is unfamiliar with you, first make sure you disclose any previous medical conditions. Hopefully, the teacher will ask you about any conditions, previous injuries, or surgeries—or even have you complete a brief survey. If not, please let the teacher know about anything that might put you at risk for injuries during the yoga class. Most teachers will appreciate this information and should be able to offer general modifications that make the sessions safer for you.

While this may seem obvious, we'll say it anyway: Yoga teachers are not doctors and are not qualified to diagnose or treat your physical ailments. Also realize that in a group setting, even the best, most educated of teachers will not be able to give everyone in class the personal attention they require. Go into the class with the attitude that you are in charge of your body, and that it is up to you to keep yourself safe. If you are unsure whether something is safe for you, decide whether you will take a risk in that moment, and then learn to live with the consequences. Or if you prefer to live more cautiously, do some research and wait until you feel you have enough knowledge to make that decision. Or modify the asana. Or just don't perform it.

In yoga class, as in the rest of life, you are responsible for yourself, so decide what is safe for you. If you are dealing with a serious health condition and considering a group class, perhaps a middle ground is to seek a yoga teacher or yoga therapist for a few private sessions so that you can better understand how to practice in a way that suits your needs.

After you have informed the teacher of your needs, drop the ego! Yoga practice is not a place for competition. As the Fishman study indicated, ego and excessive effort are the main factors that could cause an injury. Don't compare yourself to the person on the mat next to you. Furthermore, don't compare yourself to yourself. Live in the present. Don't compare yourself with what you did last year, last month, last week, or even yesterday. Sense where you are today. It could be that you can stretch a bit farther today, you may be tired and cannot go as far, or you might have had a stressful day and cannot focus on your practice. Distractions always increase the chance of injury. Pay attention to how *you* are doing, not the person on the mat next to you. This can drastically decrease your chance of injury.

The study also indicated that inadequate or improper instructions were high on the list of factors that can cause injuries. You might think this is beyond your control, but it is not. If an instruction does not make sense or if you didn't quite understand, ask for clarification. Just raise your hand and ask the teacher to come over and explain. Most teachers will appreciate your asking and will likely clarify the instruction for the whole class. It is highly unlikely that you were the only person in class who didn't understand the instruction, so the other students will appreciate an explanation too.

However, there is a fine line between asking targeted questions and being disruptive to the class. Use your judgment and be sensitive to that balance. If you find yourself in a class that leaves you with more questions than answers, then the class level or teacher might not be the right fit. Seek a different class or teacher better suited to your learning style and needs.

You can follow general guidelines to protect yourself. These safety tips are something to consider even if you have never had an injury in a specific area of your body. If you have a preexisting condition in a specific area, then it is even more important that you consider these guidelines. So let's look at specific body areas and safety tips for those areas.

Low-Back and Lumbar Spine Pain

Low-back pain, or pain in the lumbar spine, is one of the most common complaints in the Western world. Approximately 80 percent of adults in the United

States experience low back pain at some point (Rubin 2007). Usually the pain goes away by itself, and it is estimated that about half of people with low-back pain do not seek treatment. Common diagnoses include disc dysfunctions, muscle strains, repetitive strain, spondylolisthesis (displacement of a lumbar vertebra), and osteoarthritis. What most of the diagnoses have in common is that symptoms come and go. Periods free from pain are followed by acute flare-ups. For some people this can turn into chronic pain. Chronic pain is an extensive topic, and new research is changing how it is viewed. For now, we will look at how you can protect your low back while performing common poses.

Forward Bend

Many people experience increased back pain when bending forward. They might complain of soreness in the back, strain, or radiating pain and numbness going down the leg. Any time a yoga movement causes radiating pain or numbness into an extremity *stop the movement immediately*. A movement or yoga pose that causes radiating pain or numbness is a sign there may be a nerve problem. Continuing the movement that causes the pain or numbness may make the problem worse. For the lumbar spine, it is usually a forward bend of the spine or a forward bend with rotation that causes the radiating pain or numbness. A backward bend is often a better option for someone with pain and numbness coming from the low back.

Forward bend poses: Standing forward fold, seated forward fold, downward-facing dog, pigeon

Use these tips to perform safe forward bends (flexion) of the lumbar spine:

○ Tilt the pelvis forward to increase lordosis in the low back. Lumbar lordosis is the healthy curve, or arch, in the low back. Maintain that lordosis during forward bends.

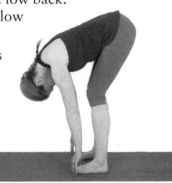

○ Spread your legs and take a wider stance. This will give you a more stable base of support.

○ Bend your knees if you have tight hamstrings (the muscles in the back of the thighs as shown in the photo) while doing forward bends. This allows your pelvis to rotate and your low back to maintain lordosis while protecting your back. When you want to stretch your hamstrings, try the reclined leg stretch variations in chapter 10.

○ Use blocks and chairs to protect your lumbar spine during forward bends. Other chapters offer suggestions on how to use these props to modify your practice.

○ Don't pull with your arms to go farther into forward bends. This increases the risk to your spine.

○ Be careful about doing any yoga pose that combines forward bending and rotation. Remember that rotation should occur in the thoracic spine (middle and upper back), not in the lumbar spine. Rotating and bending forward puts a high amount of stress on the lumbar spine, even if you don't have a preexisting condition of the low back. If you have a disc problem or another low-back dysfunction, you may want to avoid this movement, or at least to be careful with it. Poses that combine spinal flexion with rotation include rotated angle, rotated lateral angle, balancing half moon, and thread the needle.

  ○ Brace with your abdomen before bending forward. This will slightly increase the tone in your abdomen and low back so that you can maintain lordosis when you enter the bend. This is especially important if you have a preexisting condition in your low back.

This technique can be helpful whenever a pose requires abdominal stabilization. It will be particularly helpful in standing poses and core work. Learning to use intraabdominal pressure can also help protect your low back in forward bends. Conversely, a soft abdomen with a focus on easy abdominal breathing can be helpful when you are doing more relaxed work in supported postures.

EXPLORATION
Breathing With Abdominal Bracing

In yoga classes, we are often instructed to draw the navel to the spine in order to find abdominal stability. And while this can be a useful thing to do, it sometimes leaves the practitioner too focused on what is happening in the front of the body and disconnects her from maintaining stability while continuing to breathe. This exercise connects you to the inner corset of the abdominal muscles while allowing you to continue to breathe efficiently in yoga poses that demand more core stability.

1 Come into a reclined position with your knees bent and feet on the floor. Inhale into your abdomen, purposefully puffing out the low belly as you do so.

2 Retain your breath and draw everything that you have just puffed out back toward the spine as if you were bracing for someone to punch you in the gut. Use your hands to feel how the rib cage, low back, and abdomen firm up as you do so.

3 Exhale. Repeat this a few times with breath retention to get a sense of the stabilizing contraction and changes in intraabdominal pressure.

4 Once you get a sense of how to do this, try to do the same thing without holding your breath. Can you hold the abdominal contraction and move your breath focus up into the rib cage as you keep the abdomen firm?

5 To help differentiate this practice, try holding the contraction at 100, 75, 50, and 25 percent as you continue to explore moving the breath up into the rib cage. Now try breathing into the rib cage and the abdomen to find the abdominal contraction without holding your breath.

6 Once you think you have it, try applying the rib cage–focused breathing to the abdominal contraction in bridge (chapter 10), balancing table (chapter 10), prone backbend, cobra (chapter 9), and mountain pose (chapter 2).

Backward Bend

Today many people spend a large portion of their working and leisure life sitting. Sitting tends to decrease the lumbar lordosis. We often are not comfortable in everyday situations, such as laying facedown, that require lumbar extension, but many people love backward bends performed in yoga because they feel like it opens them up. While gentle backward bends are generally considered safer to perform than forward bends, some people have difficulty with backward bends because of a variety of conditions.

Backward bend poses: Standing backbend, cobra, bow, camel, bridge

Follow these tips to perform safe backward bends (extensions) of the lumbar spine:

∘ Extend the thoracic spine first. One of the keys to safe movement that will not strain the lumbar spine is to increase the mobility of the thoracic spine. Therefore, extend the thoracic spine first (as seen in the photo) before extending the lumbar spine. Brace before you go into a backward bend. Just as with forward bends, try to slightly increase the tone of your abdominal and back muscles before you begin the movement. This will help protect your lumbar spine.

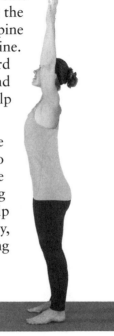

∘ Don't focus excessively on what is happening in the back of the body during backward bends. Bring the focus to the front of the body and think about creating length before bending backward. Focus on maintaining that length during the asana. Eventually you will be able to sense the relationship between what is happening in the front and back of the body, bringing them into an effective balance during your backbending practices.

∘ Although it is not as common to experience radiating leg pain or numbness during backbends, stop the movement if you experience either.

∘ Do not extend and rotate the lumbar spine at the same time. Remember that rotation happens in the thoracic spine, so ensure your middle and upper back is mobile enough to take stress off the lumbar spine before attempting to combine extension and rotation.

∘ Spondylolisthesis (a slippage of one vertebra on another) is one of the more common conditions that causes pain during backbends. A person with this condition should avoid backbends. They will usually complain of a sharp or biting pain in the low back when they extend the back or while coming up from a forward bend.

Spinal Rotations and Twists

One of the reasons that yoga practices can be effective for people with low-back pain is that many poses involve movement or rotation of the thoracic spine. As with any asana, it is important that twists be performed correctly and without excessive effort. You must be able to discern where in the spine the rotation happens, which requires awareness and mindfulness.

Rotation poses: Standing twist, seated twist, reclined twist

Here are tips for performing safe rotations of the spine:

∘ The anatomy of the lumbar spine limits rotation; therefore, rotation must occur in the thoracic spine. Make sure some of your asana practice focuses on the mobility of the thoracic spine and midback.

∘ If the thoracic spine becomes stiff, it will limit rotation and you will likely try to rotate from the lumbar spine instead, which can lead to lumbar spine injuries. Protect the lumbar spine by keeping the thoracic spine mobile.

EXPLORATION

Anchoring in Spinal Twist

1 During the seated twist, first notice your ischial tuberosities, also known as the sits bones. When you sit on something hard, you can probably feel those bony prominences that are touching the surface you are sitting on. If you have difficulty feeling them, put your hands between yourself and the seat and wiggle a bit from side to side. Now can you feel your sits bones?

2 Once you have identified the ischial tuberosities, move from side to side until you are bearing the same amount of weight on each sits bone. Now twist to either side. Make sure that you maintain equal weight and pressure on each sits bone (a). How far can you rotate your spine without shifting the weight more toward one sits bone or the other? Chances are if you are making sure you maintain equal weight on both sits bones, you are rotating using the thoracic spine and not the lumbar spine.

3 Next, twist and allow the weight to move more onto one sits bone (b). Can you feel the difference? Do you notice how you are less precise in your twist when you shift the weight onto one sits bone and how more of the rotation takes place in areas other than the thoracic spine? Limiting this imbalance can help protect your lumbar spine.

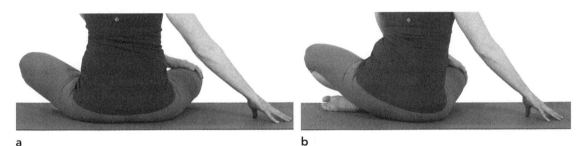

a   b

4 Similar to how you monitored your sits bones while twisting in a seated position, to safely twist while standing, balance your weight on both feet and make sure that it is equally distributed among the three points of the foot (first metatarsal head, fifth metatarsal head, and the calcaneus, or heel bone). Rotate your spine while maintaining a stable pelvis and balancing the weight on those three points on each foot. Do not shift the weight through the feet or to either side as you twist. If you are maintaining equal weight on the three points in each foot, you are rotating through the thoracic spine and not the lumbar spine. Now twist while letting the weight shift more onto one foot and sense how that changes where the spinal rotation takes place.

The feedback you get from your body, the sits bones, and the feet will allow you to determine whether you are rotating from the thoracic spine or from somewhere else. Of course, you have to accept that you will not be able to rotate as far when you move safely, but as mentioned in the *Bhagavad Gita*, "Yoga is skillful action." To move with precision is a skill. You can move farther if you move without precision, but you increase the risk of injury if you use unskilled movements.

Neck and Cervical Spine

The cervical spine allows more general mobility in all directions than either the thoracic or lumbar spine. Just like with the lumbar spine, many of the dysfunctions of the cervical spine can be relieved by increasing the mobility of the thoracic spine. Less research has been conducted on cervical spine dysfunction than on lumbar spine dysfunction. Many of the problems, such as disc dysfunction and muscle strain, that occur in the lumbar spine also occur in the cervical spine. As we pointed out when discussing the lumbar spine, yoga poses should not cause radiating pain or numbness. If that occurs, modify or stop the pose to avoid causing pain or numbness.

Cervical spine poses: Cobra, bow, camel, standing twist, seated twist, bridge, warrior 2

Follow these tips to protect the cervical spine during common asanas:

∘ Extend the thoracic spine before you extend the cervical spine (see photo below). Any time an asana calls for cervical extension, make sure that you also extend the thoracic spine. Sense the lengthening in the front of the body when you extend the neck. You do not want to jackknife the neck and move only the lower part of it when you extend the cervical spine. When performing a cervical extension, try to keep length in the back of the neck and resist the urge to collapse the head back toward the shoulder blades.

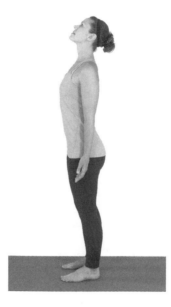

∘ Align the neck and head with the rest of the spine. In any asana, especially in asanas requiring rotation, keep the cervical spine and head aligned with the rest of the spine (as shown in the photo). It is easy to overrotate the cervical spine to compensate for decreased mobility in the thoracic area.

∘ Retract the chin straight in toward the throat, and extend the upper cervical spine during the poses. This prevents the head-forward posture during asanas.

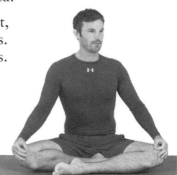

◦ Avoid fully extending and rotating the cervical spine. Combining extension and rotation of the neck can pinch the structures coming out of the cervical spine. This isn't a big risk, but why take a chance?

Follow these tips to protect the cervical spine during inversions:

◦ Only do inversions that you are comfortable with and that you have practiced. Don't try to do full inversions such as shoulder stands or head stands right away, if ever.

◦ Start slowly. Lying with the legs up the wall or even putting a block under the pelvis might be enough of an inversion.

◦ We have intentionally left shoulder stand and plow out of our pose explorations because properly explaining the biomechanical differences required for safety is too complicated for this format. We find that postures that offer the potential for loaded cervical flexion (shoulder stand, plow) and weight bearing in the cervical spine (certain variations of head a stand) have a higher risk-to-reward ratio than other poses, and for that reason we have left them out of this book. If you want to learn those postures, we highly recommend working one on one with a yoga teacher or yoga therapist who is skilled at biomechanical assessments and can offer you nuanced, progressive, and personalized instruction.

Shoulders and Upper Extremities

In yoga practice, the shoulders and upper extremities are asked to do something they normally don't do: bear weight. Normally, we hold weight only on the lower extremities, and anatomically the lower extremities are built for stability, locomotion, and weight bearing. The upper extremities, on the other hand, are built for mobility and relationships with others. We reach out to others to give or receive using our upper extremities. In asanas, such as downward-facing dog, cat, cow, and table, we bear weight on the upper extremities. Not only are we asked to bear weight on the upper extremities, but we are also asked to move through the full range of motion (ROM) of the shoulders in overhead movements. Most of us do not go through the full ROM of our shoulders during daily activities. We probably don't even raise our arms above shoulder height or 90 degrees. Then in yoga class we raise our arms overhead and may also bear weight on them when they are almost at the end ROM. No wonder some people complain of sore shoulders after a yoga session.

Shoulder poses: Standing crescent moon, gate, side plank, table, plank, downward-facing dog, warrior 1

Follow these tips to protect the shoulders during asanas:

◦ Align the shoulders with the elbows and wrists. Determine where you feel the most stable when bearing weight on the upper extremities.

◦ Use your core muscles to pull away from the floor as you stabilize your arms and push your hands into the floor. You need stability in the shoulder blades and the central core in order to be able to protect the upper extremities in an asana.

◦ The sense of stability comes from the shoulder blades. Set the shoulder blades before you start full weight bearing on the upper extremities. In general, you should hold the shoulder blades slightly down and in toward the thoracic spine.

Shoulder Stabilization

1 In a facedown position, place your forehead on a rolled-up towel. Arms are by your sides and slightly away from the body with the palms facing up.

2 Keep your upper back and neck relaxed as you squeeze the bottom of the scapulas down the back, then in toward each other as you lift your arms off of the ground. Hold for a count of five. Repeat three times.

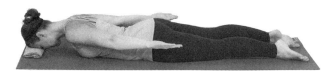

3 Starting in the same facedown position, bring the arms to shoulder height in a goal-post shape with the palms on the ground. Keep your upper back and neck relaxed as you squeeze the bottom of the scapulas down the back and then in toward each other as you lift the arms off the ground and draw the bent elbows in toward the body. Hold for a count of five. Repeat three times.

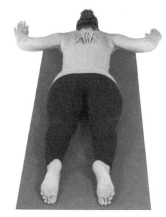

4 Starting in the same facedown position, extend the arms straight in front of you with the palms down on the ground. Keep your upper back and neck relaxed as you squeeze the bottom of the scapulas down the back and then in toward each other as you lift the arms off the ground. Hold for a count of five. Repeat three times.

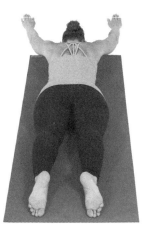

If you find that you cannot control the shoulder blades in a particular asana, then the pose is too advanced for you and you need more strength and control in the muscles moving the shoulder blades. Without the stable platform of the shoulder blades, you run an increased risk of injuring the shoulders, elbows, and wrists. Skilled action of the shoulder blades requires controlled mobility.

Elbows

The elbow is a fairly stable joint and is not often injured in yoga. The main problem is too much movement in the elbow—that is hyperextending the elbow (bending it backward).

Elbow poses: Side plank, table, plank, downward-facing dog

Follow these tips to protect the elbows during asanas:

○ Don't hyperextend the elbow. If you have this ability, it may be tempting to hyperextend if it feels easier to hold the asana. The problem is that you are "hanging" on the elbow ligaments and the ligaments will likely become increasingly lax. Also when you hang on the ligaments, the muscles are not engaged, so if you lose your balance, it might take longer to find it, causing you to fall and hurt your shoulder, spine, or other vulnerable places.

○ Learning to avoid hyperextension starts with microbending the elbow, and keeping the insides of the elbows forward as you gently traction the heels of the hands back toward the hips without actually moving them. From this position, you can start to find the shoulder-stabilizing muscles and learn to avoid hanging from the ligaments.

Wrists

Many of us are spending more and more time working on computers or typing on our phones. We use our fingers to perform very small movements over and over. Couple that with a more sedentary lifestyle and it is no wonder we see an increase in the number of people with carpal tunnel syndrome and other wrist problems. Any kind of weight bearing through the upper extremities might increase the pain in the wrists and hands, but weight bearing through the upper extremities can also be a wonderful opportunity to alleviate wrist and hand problems.

Wrist poses: Side plank, table, plank, downward-facing dog

Follow these tips to protect the wrists during asanas:

○ Most of the tips we suggested under the shoulder section also apply to the wrist, especially the information about stability and controlled mobility of the shoulder blades. If the shoulder blades are unstable, then the muscles of the shoulders and the smaller muscles of the forearm have to work to keep the arms stable and aligned. This will quickly lead to overuse of the forearms and wrists. So maintain strength and stability of the shoulder blades to avoid overworking the wrists and forearms during asana practice.

○ Keep the rib cage mobile, the chin tucked in, and the arm pits open. This will ensure that you don't close off blood or lymph vessels to the hands and that the nerves will not be compromised on their way to the hands.

° If you experience pain in the wrists, numbness, or tingling, modify the pose. Instead of putting weight on the hands, bend your elbows, and put the weight on the forearms. You can also avoid putting full weight on the arms by changing the orientation or doing a pose against the wall (*a*). Start slowly and progress toward full weight bearing (*b*). Yoga can do wonders for people with wrist pain, but they have to modify the poses as needed or their symptoms could worsen.

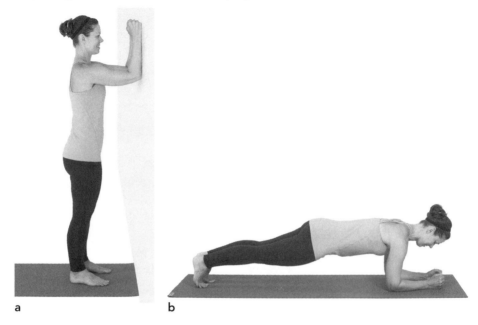

a   b

Hips and Lower Extremities

Compared to the upper extremities, which are built for mobility and relationships, the lower extremities are built for weight bearing, locomotion, and stability. The problem with the hips is that they tend to be too stable. We lose mobility and end up with arthritis and other problems, eventually leading to surgery, hip replacements, or problems in the knees, ankles, and feet. In addition, the angle that the head of the femur (the ball of the ball-and-socket hip joint) connects to the pelvis can vary greatly. This means there is a vast person-to-person difference in hip mobility. This partly has to do with how the lower extremities develop.

Hip poses: Bow, camel, gate, warrior 1, warrior 2, triangle, yoga squat, pigeon, frog

Follow these tips to protect the hips during asanas:

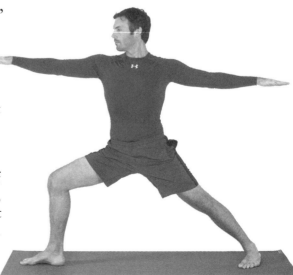

° Take instructions about the correct foot placement in standing poses, such as warrior, with a grain of salt. The amount that your foot can turn out or in depends on your skeletal structure. Instead of placing your foot at a specific angle, sense where all three parts of the foot bear weight equally and where you feel stability and strength through the leg to the spine and out through the arms.

° Learn to differentiate the hip from the pelvis. In a standing position, can you turn the hip without turning the pelvis? Can you turn the pelvis without turning the hip? Can you move the pelvis and hip as a single unit? These nuanced movements allow you to differentiate and explore your own safety and stability.

° Try keeping your "hip pit" open. The hip pit is the area in the front of the hip that folds when you bend the hip to take a step forward. As with the armpit, the hip pit has vessels and nerves running through it, and to maintain freedom of the hip, this area should stay open.

° Engage the glutes. The large gluteal muscles produce power. Most people do not put themselves in situations where they have to use lots of power to extend the hips. Instead they use the hamstrings. You know if you are engaging the hamstrings instead of the glutes if your hamstrings cramp while you are bridging. Try to engage the glutes first. Your hamstrings will thank you.

EXPLORATION
Activating the Glutes

❶ From a facedown position, place your hands on top of each other and let your forehead rest on them. Bend the knees and flex the feet. Keeping equal weight in the front of the pelvis, squeeze the left buttock to lift the lower part of the thigh off of the ground and slowly lower it back down. Focus on control and glute activation rather than height. Repeat on the right side. Alternate side to side for a count of 10 on each side (a).

❷ From a facedown position, place your hands on top of each other and let your forehead rest on them. Bend the knees and bring them out toward the edge of the mat with the heels touching. Squeeze the glutes to lift the knees and the lower part of the thighs off of the floor. Hold for 5 seconds and repeat five times (b).

❸ From a facedown position, place your hands on top of each other and let your forehead rest on them. Extend the legs straight behind you. Initiate the action of lifting the left leg by focusing on the place where the bottom of the buttock meets the upper thigh. Repeat on the right side. Alternate side to side for a count of 10 on each side (c).

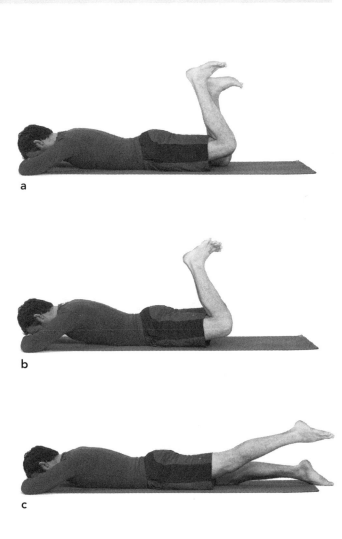

a

b

c

Knees

As mentioned previously, many people experience limited mobility and rotation of the hips. When the ability to rotate the hips is limited and the feet are anchored to the ground in a certain placement, the only other option for rotation is in the knees. Although the knee allows some rotational movement, it is primarily a hinge that flexes and extends. When people experience decreased rotational ability in the hips, many try to rotate in the knees more than is possible. This can eventually lead to meniscus injuries and increased wear and tear.

Knee poses: Seated twist, warrior 1, warrior 2, triangle, yoga squat, pigeon, frog

Follow these tips to protect the knees during asanas:

○ In standing poses, align the knee close to the area over the first and second toe. In most standing poses, the knee should not extend in front of the foot. If you cannot maintain that knee position, the asana is too difficult for you. Avoid going too deep into the pose.

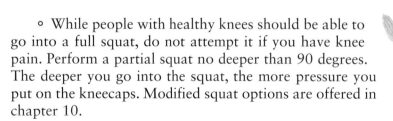

○ While people with healthy knees should be able to go into a full squat, do not attempt it if you have knee pain. Perform a partial squat no deeper than 90 degrees. The deeper you go into the squat, the more pressure you put on the kneecaps. Modified squat options are offered in chapter 10.

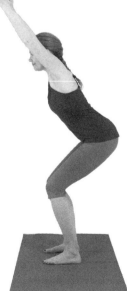

○ Narrow the stance in standing poses if you have knee pain. This puts less pressure on the kneecaps and joints.

○ Center the foot over the three points of contact to find grounding and establish stability. The more stability and balance you can find from below, the better the knees will be aligned.

○ Don't hyperextend the knee. Many people are drawn to yoga because they are very flexible. Just as with hyperextension of the elbow, it is easy to hang on the ligaments in the knee and not engage the leg muscles. The risk is that you will stretch the ligaments and joint capsule even more if you lose your balance while the muscles are disengaged, and you are more likely to fall. Learning to avoid hyperextending the knee joint starts with microbending the knee and bringing the shin forward as you pull the thigh back. From this position, you can start to find the quadriceps muscles and learn to avoid hanging in your ligaments.

Feet and Ankles

The feet and ankles take a lot of abuse from the shoes we wear and the surfaces on which we walk. Your feet should be able to adapt to different surfaces and shoes. Your ability to sense yourself in space (proprioception) depends a lot on input from the feet and ankles. It has been said that we die from the ground up. Once a person starts to lose touch with the feet and tighten the ankles, the risk of falling increases and other areas of the body start tightening as well. This further increases the risk of falling and in response, the person limits his or her activities. It is a vicious cycle to be avoided. For many people, the yoga studio may be the only place where they go barefoot, and they might therefore feel insecure and wobbly.

Foot and ankle poses: Child's pose, gate, side plank, bridge, downward-facing dog, mountain, tree, warrior 1, warrior 2, triangle, yoga squat

Follow these tips to protect the feet and ankles during asanas:

Evenly distribute your weight among the three points of the foot: the head of the first metatarsal (bone behind big toe), the head of the fifth metatarsal (the bone behind the little toe), and the calcaneus (heel bone). Your balance is greatly improved when the weight is evenly distributed among these points. To maintain this equilibrium, pay attention to the information you receive from your feet.

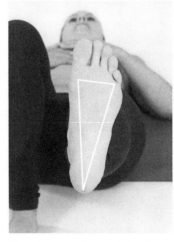

The three points of the foot.

○ If you have poor balance, stand next to a wall. If you are unaccustomed to being shoeless and feel like shoes will improve your balance, then bring a pair of clean shoes to the yoga studio and wear them. Hopefully, with time, you can train yourself to be comfortable barefoot while practicing yoga and walking around your home.

○ Slowly swaying from side to side as part of your warm-up before a yoga session can also increase foot awareness and improve balance.

After reading about yoga injuries and how to prevent them, you might be wondering "Is yoga a good choice for me?" After all, people are breaking legs, hurting shoulders, and so on. Well, the good news is that yoga is relatively safe, and you control most of the risks. Don't let the ego take over and tempt you to compete with your neighbor. Inform the teacher about your medical concerns. If you don't understand instructions, ask for clarification. Most important, be aware of how you move and what feels secure. Use your practice to learn how to pay attention and respond to both obvious and subtle bodily feedback. Challenge yourself, but only within the limits of what you consider safe.

EXPLORATION

Tennis Ball Foot Rolling

This exercise can be done standing or seated. It is intended to wake up and release tension in the feet. Depending on your personal history, you may find places in your feet that make you say "holy cow" or another expression of surprised intensity. This is fairly normal for most people. If the pressure is too much, back off of the body weight that you put onto the foot from standing, or do the exercise from a seated position in a chair to reduce intensity. If you have challenges with balance, you can do the exercise standing next to a wall and steady yourself with one hand.

❶ Grab a tennis ball or any ball of a similar size that is firm but slightly pliable. To get a baseline for how you experience your feet, stand in mountain pose (chapter 2) and tree pose (chapter 10) and pay attention to how your feet connect to the ground. From the ground, follow the pathway of connection from your foot through the knee into the hip, pelvis, spine, and core.

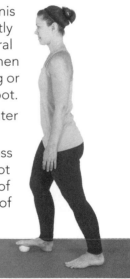

❷ From mountain, place one foot slightly behind you. Place a tennis ball under the ball of the front foot under the big toe mound. Gently lean into the front foot to put pressure on the tennis ball. Do this several times in a pulsing motion, leaning in with your body weight and then backing off. You can control the intensity of the sensation by lessening or increasing how much body weight you put onto the ball of the front foot.

❸ Repeat this action as you move the ball slowly across to the center of the ball of the foot and then over to the pinky toe side.

❹ Move the ball to the mid foot, continuing to work your way across while repeating the same pulsing action. Be gentle with the mid foot as you will encounter some tendons there. Finish by moving the ball of the foot onto the ground and placing the tennis ball under the heel of the foot. Finish with the big toe side of the heel, the center, and the pinky toe side.

❺ When you are finished with the first foot, revisit mountain and tree pose (on both feet) to see how your feet connect to the ground, comparing the foot and leg that was released to the one that hasn't yet received the release.

❻ When you are ready, repeat on the other foot.

Staying Injury Free in Any Activity

Now that you've learned to avoid injuries during your yoga practice, we'll discuss how your yoga practice can help you avoid injuries in the rest of your life. We will not be so bold as to guarantee an injury-free, active life if you play with and explore our concepts. But we will make the bold statement that you can increase your chance of avoiding injuries while performing any chosen activity if you play with variations and explorations. We won't examine how to use the concepts in this book for individual activities because there are countless activities that people enjoy. Instead we will group activities into categories, discussing yoga's benefit to activities from each category. You can then look at the activities you like to perform, see which category fits, and get ideas about how the explorations in this book might translate to the performance of your chosen activity. Some activities might fall into multiple categories.

Endurance, or Linear, Activities

Typical endurance activities include running, walking, swimming, and biking. Although your opponents might be faster or have more endurance, you usually don't have to respond to their unexpected moves. You can perform the activity by yourself and occasionally enter a race to see if you have improved. These endurance activities are linear and repetitive. A runner or walker takes about 2,000 steps in a mile (1.6 km), and the majority of those steps are similar. If you walk or run on an uneven surface, your stride length and how your foot lands will vary, but generally the first step is similar to the next step, and the next, and so on. Other endurance activities, such as swimming and cycling, are similar in that you repeat the same movement over and over with little variation.

Remember, nerves that fire together wire together. The nervous system likes to perform movements in a familiar manner because that is the most efficient way it has figured out how to perform the movement based on the available information. There's nothing wrong with that unless you get hurt or are using certain parts of your body more than others in an asymmetrical way. Your injuries in linear activities are generally of the overuse type, and you can focus on how you perform the repetitive movement and how you have compensated for old injuries or habits in order to avoid injuries.

If you have ever been injured, you know that your whole body adapts to the injury. You move in ways that make you hurt less. If possible, you continue to do the same activities as always, including endurance activities. Your nervous system arranges or organizes the body so that you

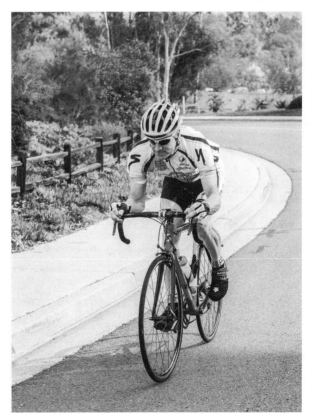

Yoga therapy concepts of play and exploration can make you more efficient during endurance activities.

© Human Kinetics

117

can move with the least amount of pain. This is how our intelligent bodies work. Our nervous systems always organize parts of our bodies so that we can perform tasks efficiently, with as little pain and discomfort as possible. The problem is that once injuries have healed, the nervous system does not suddenly realize, "Oh, this body part has healed. Now let's go back to the pre-injury body organization." No, the nervous system more than likely continues to protect you against an injury that is no longer there, and after weeks or months, this becomes your new normal. For an endurance athlete, this new normal likely means that unequal wear and tear is put on the left and right sides of the body. After years of this new normal, osteoarthritis or other chronic injuries start to appear with increasing frequency.

Remember the quote in chapter 3 by Moshe Feldenkrais: "If you don't know what you are doing, you can't do what you want." Well if you don't know that you are compensating for an injury that has healed, you can't correct the way you are performing the activity. By using the concepts of identification, differentiation, and integration, you will increase your awareness of what you are doing and you can notice how you are performing your endurance activity. If you play with these concepts when you are recovering from an injury, your nervous system will recognize when it is safe to go back to the body organization you had before the injury happened. In this way, you will avoid falling into chronically compensating movement patterns. If you have already fallen into patterns of compensation based on an old injury, the concepts presented in this book will help you recognize those patterns. You can then differentiate the compensated pattern to find your way to a more varied and efficient one.

Even if you are lucky enough to have never had an injury, the concepts presented in this book can help you in your endurance activities. You can explore and play to learn more efficient ways to breathe and use your lungs. If you are a runner, you might find out that you are not pushing off from the ground efficiently. If you are a cyclist, you might realize that you are only pushing down on the pedal and not using the cleats to pull up during the back of the pedal stroke, thereby losing power. If you swim, you might discover that you use the left and right arms differently or that by playing with how the hand moves through the water your stroke is more efficient. The possibilities to adjust, adapt, and improve your endurance activity are endless.

Agility, or Nonlinear, Activities

Activities that require you to respond to unexpected moves and events are more unpredictable than straight-line endurance activities. Therefore, the focus of your yoga practice will be somewhat different. Whether the activity is basketball, tennis, volleyball, or any other activity where you compete against another person, responding to his moves, our approach to yoga therapy can greatly increase the skills you need to enjoy these kinds of sports.

In nonlinear activities, such as basketball, you will try to outmaneuver your opponent while she is trying to outmaneuver you. In tennis you are trying to place the ball where the opponent cannot reach and she is trying to do the same to you. These kinds of activities are unpredictable. You will not always be in the ideal position to hit or catch the ball or defend against the opponent. For these kinds of activities, the differentiation aspect, especially in the transition phase, can not only yield large benefits in helping you stay injury free, but also allow you to outsmart your opponent.

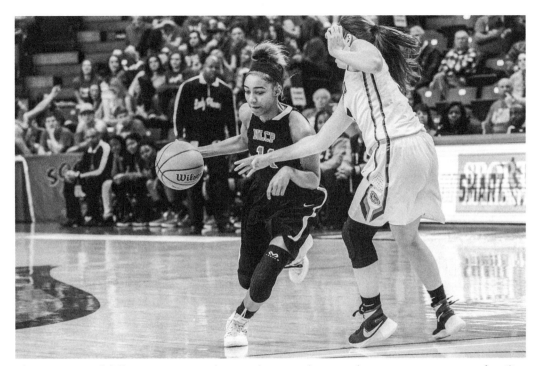

The concept of differentiation can be used to avoid injury when you assume an unfamiliar position during agility sports.

© Human Kinetics

As with the endurance activities, using the concepts of identification, differentiation, and integration can prevent injuries in unpredictable, nonlinear activities. We talked about how the nervous system likes to solve puzzles. In the case of these nonlinear sports, the nervous system needs to learn to recognize positions when the proprioceptors are not lined up. Do I know where my feet are when I cut left or right? Do I know how to hit when my head is turned away from the ball, or catch the ball when my arms and head are pointing in different directions? If your nervous system does not recognize these positions or is not adaptable enough to respond to these positions, then your muscles will not react as quickly and the result might be a muscle strain or ligament sprain. By playing with differentiations on and off the mat, the nervous system learns to recognize more body organizations, thereby increasing the flexibility and adaptability of the nervous system and leading to a decreased injury risk when you are in an imperfect position. So instead of being overly concerned about overuse injuries, as you are with linear and endurance activities, here you are more concerned about injuries that happen in body organizations that the nervous system does not recognize.

To teach your nervous system to handle these situations, try to focus more on the transitions. How can you transition between asanas in different ways? When the tennis ball or basketball is coming toward you at full speed, you are likely moving while you hit or catch the ball. Using the language of yoga, you can say that at the moment you hit or catch the ball you are performing the asana. But between catching or hitting, you are transitioning to prepare for the next asana, hit, or catch. By varying and paying attention to transitions during your asana practice, your nervous system is getting used to various ways of going from one asana to the next. This makes the nervous system more adaptable and, with some practice on the court, you will be more efficient and less injury prone when going from asana to asana on the court.

You can also play with this concept by stringing together sequences in different ways. If you always go from warrior 1 to warrior 2 and then to mountain, try going from warrior 2 straight into tree pose or some other pose that doesn't typically follow warrior 2. Or you can go into tree between warrior 1 and 2. We are not suggesting you do this all the time, but if you are looking at injury prevention in nonlinear activities, you need to challenge the nervous system by doing things in unexpected ways. That is, give the nervous system new puzzles to solve. In activities such as basketball, tennis, and volleyball, where players make unpredictable, nonlinear moves, you need to train the nervous system for the unpredictable if you want to decrease your chances of injuries.

Another benefit for people who enjoy nonlinear activities is that they will become better at what they are doing. Not only will they enjoy their activities more, but by using the ideas in this book they will also become better at them. By identifying your favorite moves on the court, and then differentiating and integrating, you will become more flexible in how you return the ball or from what positions you can shoot, for example.

Everyday Activities

Here we consider all the activities you do during the day. Look at an activity that you want to improve, that causes pain, that you want to enjoy more, or that you want to start doing. Decide whether the activity is more linear or nonlinear. If it is more linear, focus on how you do the activity or asana. Are you compensating somewhere for old injuries? Do you have the strength and flexibility needed to maintain the organization of your body to do that activity over and over in the same manner? How else could you perform the activity or asana? What if in warrior 1 you turned your back foot a different way or turned your pelvis differently? Did that change the way you then performed your activity? In chapters 9 and 10 we introduce lots of variations for some asanas. If you have other asanas that you prefer, can you use the examples in those chapters and apply some of those ideas to your favorite asanas—or even better, to your favorite linear activities?

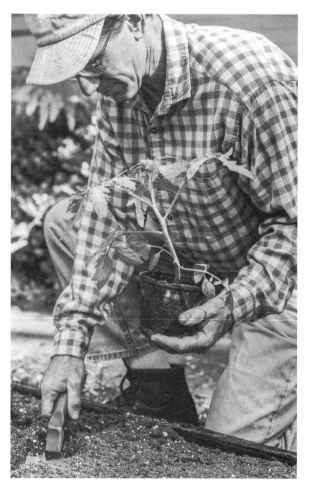

Many everyday activities, such as gardening, are a blend of linear and nonlinear movements.

If the everyday activity that you want to improve is more of the nonlinear type, then play with the ideas outlined for nonlinear activities. Play more with the transition between asanas. Perform the transitions in different ways. Change the sequence of your practice from day to day. Play with how you transition during this nonlinear, everyday activity. How can you go from one activity to the next in different ways? These are examples of ways to use the concepts of identification, differentiation, and integration to avoid injuries during your activities and to become better at how you do them.

Please note that how you use the concepts in this book depends on your intention. Much of what we have presented is geared toward giving you a more flexible, robust, and adaptable nervous system that will allow you to stay active throughout your life. If your intention is to calm the nervous system or to develop focus, then you will not differentiate as much. You will likely slow your movements or hold an asana longer, with your focus on the messages emerging from your body. Although those practices and intentions are just as valuable as the practices we have introduced in this book, that is not our focus. Our focus here is to allow you to stay active without injuries, enjoying those activities for the remainder of your life.

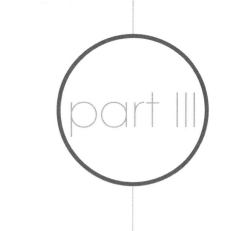

part III

Poses for Lifelong Fitness

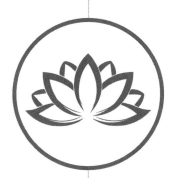

eight
Intentions and Connections

Yoga therapy offers paths and perspectives from which you can inquire into your relationships with yourself, others, and the greater whole. Fully exploring your potential for awareness and realization could fill several lifetimes of inquiry. Yet awareness is an interesting thing, particularly when you try to gain more of it. How can you go about making conscious that which is unconscious? Yoga therapy offers structures to observe your thoughts, beliefs, and habits. When you use your yoga practice to bring awareness to previously unexamined aspects of yourself, you have the opportunity to make what was previously an unconscious choice a conscious one. This experimentation with awareness and intention can change your experience of yoga practice and the activities of daily life.

EXPLORATION
The Effect of Your Thoughts on Your Body

❶ Stand in mountain pose. Determine the baseline for how you are feeling right now. Start by noticing how your body has organized itself in standing upright. You can do this by observing skeletal relationships—noticing where your feet are in relationship to your pelvis; where your pelvis is in relationship to your spine and feet; where your spine is in relationship to the feet and head; and where your head is in relationship to your feet, pelvis, and spine. Notice your breath in a natural state without attempting to change it. Tune into the rhythm of your heartbeat.

❷ Now think of someone or something in your life that is negative or think of a past experience that was painful. Notice how your body reorganizes itself in response to this negative input. Check in with all aspects from the previous step to see what changed.

❸ Go back to mountain pose. Now think of someone or something that gives you hope or inspiration or of a past experience that gave you tremendous joy. Notice how your body reorganizes itself in response to this positive input, again using the checkpoints from step 1 and any other observations.

❹ Now pick an exercise, any exercise you like. You can try something simple such as picking up something heavy off the ground like a basket of laundry. Think of the negative memory and do the exercise. If you are using the laundry basket, pick it up and put it back down. Repeat the same actions with the positive memory in mind.

Did this exercise help you see that your thoughts carry potent energy? Did you notice that the exercise or act of lifting was better supported by your positive thoughts than the negative ones? Your thoughts can create a substantial part of your perception of reality. When you start to gain clarity about how your thoughts affect your life experience, you can choose your thoughts more consciously through the practice of awareness and intention. The power of intention can support and enhance all activities of life.

What Is Intention?

Intention is simply the act of naming why you are doing something. It answers these questions: For what purpose? With what attitude? In what way? Intention typically forms the foundation of a more superficial goal. For example, a goal may be to firm your abs, and the intentions associated with that might be to support spinal health, to become more proficient at kung fu, or to balance the energy at your solar plexus.

When people practice yoga, their intentions are as unique as they are. Take breathing for example, the lungs inflate (to different levels of efficiency) regardless of where you attempt to direct your breath. However, if your intention is to breathe into the rib cage, typically the sensation of the rib cage expanding with inhalation and contracting with exhalation is more pronounced. If you intend to explore the energy of your heart in practice, that will create a different type of experience, such as a potent sense of the heart beating, warmth in the chest, or a greater sense of lightness in the body.

Engaging with different styles of yoga produces a variety of experiences or intentions, some of which will resonate with you more than others. Usually when people say they like a particular style of yoga, it means that they are consciously or unconsciously aligned with the intention of the style or the teacher's personal intention for the classes that they are sharing.

In both ancient and modern times, people have gotten caught up in polarizing arguments about how one style or intention for practice is better than another. Our perspective is that yoga is vast and can contain a multitude of intentions. It is imperative for practitioners to identify their *own* intentions for practice in order to be empowered. From this place of careful consideration, it becomes much easier to create a clear and purposeful personal relationship with yoga therapy practices.

In yoga classes, it is often suggested that practitioners set an intention at the beginning of practice, but the process of how to set one that is appropriate for your personal needs isn't always fully explored. It can be helpful to think of intention as the motivating factor, purpose, or will behind an action. Intention sets the potent energy of your thoughts into action, creating some of the causes and effects that determine your experience of life. When you come to your yoga mat, intention directs your experience of practice. A sequence of poses is just a couple of shapes strung together, and that is all that it would ever be were it not for the intention of the teacher or practitioner. Without the marriage of individual intention with breath, yoga poses could be nothing more than glorified calisthenics. Yet when we embody a pose with a clear intention, it becomes a union of action and purpose. This union of action and purpose means that the potential intentions available for practice are as multidimensional and varied as the human experience.

Setting an Intention

1 Take a moment to consider why you are reading this book. What motivated you to pick it up in the first place? What keeps you reading? How has what you have learned so far supported your goals for living an active lifestyle?

2 Ask yourself what goals you have for creating a personalized yoga therapy practice? This might take time to narrow down, but as you do so, try to be as specific as possible in naming the goal.

3 Once you have named your goal, inquire into why it is important for you to achieve it. Keep on asking yourself "why" until you uncover a meaningful virtue that connects you with a strong sense of purpose. See whether you can narrow it down to just one word or concept. When you find it, write it down.

4 Apply the concept or word to your yoga therapy practices. See whether it resonates immediately or needs to be refined over time. Revisit the previous steps if necessary until you find an intention that supports and uplifts as you continue to pursue your goals.

It is common when we first start practicing yoga that our intentions might lean toward the superficial over the spiritual. We're only human, and the desire to look and feel good motivates us to do some awesome (and sometimes less-than-awesome) things. It's tempting to demean superficial motivations such as developing "rock-hard abs" or a "yoga butt" as being of lesser value, but these desires are real, and we have to work with them as a starting point. I (Kristen) started practicing yoga as a stressed-out twentysomething struggling with the transition to an office job from the restaurant business. My body was accustomed to moving all day long, and after a year of being stuck at a desk, I gained weight and felt uncomfortable in my body for the first time in my life. Yoga seemed like the easiest way to move my body and lose some weight. If someone had told me back then that my weight-loss intention for practice would change over time into something more meaningful or deeper, I probably would have told them to place their sanctimonious notions where the sun doesn't shine.

Luckily, I had skillful teachers who guided my practice in a way that allowed me to slowly uncover the powerful virtues hidden within my superficial goal. My deeper intentions for losing weight ended up being about creating healthier work–life boundaries and taking better care of myself. Eventually, those intentions started to relate to the bigger picture of my life's purpose and led me to become a yoga therapist. Of course, my path is unique and won't be the same as yours, but it highlights how an intention can evolve over time when you use what you learn through practice to connect the dots between your desires and goals and the virtues that are hidden within them.

Making Connections

One of the most challenging things about a yoga pose is that many of its important experiences are internal. It can be challenging to offer guidance for an internal experience. Guiding an individual practitioner toward uncovering the varied potentials of practice is more a process of inquiring than it is a set of techniques or bullet points. It is an art form.

Yoga offers the structure of the koshas, or layers, as a guide for inquiring into and making connections between the five qualities of being. They include the physical, energetic, emotional, mental, and spiritual aspects of the human experience. More than just an esoteric concept, the koshas are aspects of yourself that you can sense and feel. When you create awareness of the koshas through intentional practice, you become more capable of consciously refining your sense of self and experience.

EXPLORATION

Sensing the Layers: Gross to Subtle

Start either lying in a comfortable reclined position or seated upright. Do your best to cultivate an attitude of curiosity and kindness toward yourself and your experience in the present moment.

❶ Physical layer. Scan your body with the intention of cultivating physical awareness. Start by paying attention to how you are lying on the ground. Notice the points of contact between your body and the floor. Notice how firm or light those points of contact are. Now notice the parts of the body that are not in contact with the floor. Imagine yourself lying on a balance beam. To which side of the beam would you be more likely to fall? Make note of what you noticed.

Now bring your attention to your feet and slowly work your way up the body until you reach the crown of the head. Pay attention to places where you feel tense or relaxed and places where you feel restricted or at ease. Notice areas of heat or coolness, or areas that are calling out for attention or movement. Notice places that you feel disconnected from. Notice spots that you are hyper aware of. Do some places "talk to you" more than others? Make a note of what you perceived.

❷ Energetic, or breath, layer. Pay attention to your natural breathing rhythm. Can you sense the movement of your breath in certain places in your body? Can you use your breath awareness to become more aware of your energy level in general? If you close your eyes, do you see colors or images associated with the breath? Do parts of the body feel alive and full of vitality or feel depleted and in need of nourishment? How do those things relate to the awareness from the physical body layer? Make note of what you noticed.

❸ Emotional layer. Scan your emotional state. Start with the more obvious and immediate emotions that come up, but also give yourself time to see whether underlying emotions are waiting to bubble up and be recognized. Is there a relationship between your sense of breath, or energy, and your emotional state? How is your emotional state reflected in your physical body? Make note of your perceptions.

❹ Mental layer. Shift your attention to your quality of mind. Is the mind busy and distracted or settled and focused? Perhaps the mind is somewhere between those extremes. If so, where? Do you experience a sense of clarity in your thoughts or confusion? Is there a sense of inner knowing? Make note of what you noticed.

❺ Spiritual layer. Now pay attention to whether you can feel yourself as part of a larger whole. Do you sense a connection to something larger than yourself? Are you inspired by this connection? If you cannot sense it, do you feel apathetic, fragmented, or disconnected in some way? This layer might be a little more difficult to notice because many people relate it to their religious beliefs, which can either block awareness or provide the structures that help cultivate it. Make a note of what you noticed.

Now see whether you can connect those five layers. Take a moment to review how or whether the layers relate to one another. How can you work more skillfully with these types of awareness in asana practice as well as in daily life?

We hope your exploration of the koshas has given you more of a sense of the layers of being and now you feel empowered to make connections between the physical, energetic, emotional, mental, and spiritual aspects of your experience. Did you notice that your awareness follows your attention?

Attention and awareness can be connected for a powerful and meaningful asana practice. As you introduce a variety of experiences to the physical body, correlating shifts will occur in your energetic, emotional, mental, or spiritual awareness. The opposite is also true: If you make a differentiation in an energetic, emotional, mental, or spiritual intention, the physical body will reorganize itself (subtly or obviously) in response to that change. This means that you can introduce new intentions through the mind or through the body. The beauty of both approaches is that one is not whole without the other. It really doesn't matter whether you go after it from the mind or from the body. What is important is that you are able to gain a better understanding of the relationships between them and how they affect your experience of life.

Your yoga therapy practices become more comprehensive when they help you deconstruct and work skillfully with the layers of being you encounter in the human experience. While we are only scratching the surface of the potential of the koshas here, we certainly hope you use what you learn in your physical practice as a catalyst to explore other aspects of yourself.

Putting It Into Practice

We organized the asana section of this book to be a user-friendly learning guide. Our intent is that you explore a variety of experiences during each pose and choose which ones support the personal intentions you create for practice. As you engage with the materials, notice that each pose starts with a set of basic instructions that lay the foundation from which you can explore the other five categories of physical intention that we have set up: basic adaptations, mobility, strength, balance, and recovery. Many pose experiences could be assigned to more than one category. In those instances, we have done our best to connect the specifics of the instructions to the type of differentiation that the pose is meant to engender. Elements of one category will often be found in another. Enjoy making those connections as you explore!

Overview of the Asana Differentiation Categories

Basic options

This category offers ways to adapt the basic pose to accommodate your body type. For some practitioners, the alternatives will be necessary in order to better accommodate underlying structural nuances, injuries, or levels of fitness that might inhibit you from doing the foundational pose. Even if you are not inhibited in the foundational pose, these options may also help you identify habits you may have developed when performing a particular pose. Exploring a variety of experiences will fine-tune your sense of them, and as your practice evolves, you will become more skilled at selecting the options that are best suited for any given need or intention you might have.

Beyond the poses, you can relate the concept of adaptability to daily life by noticing how you react to different life situations. What are your patterns of habitual response to the more mundane activities of daily life? Are they the same on the mat as they are off the mat? Can you "try on" different thought patterns or perspectives throughout the day? How does adapting your breathing patterns or internal dialogue or exploring nuances in your emotional range change your experience of common life situations?

Mobility

The options in this category focus on developing your ability to differentiate joint actions in a particular pose. One of the major misconceptions people have about yoga is that it is all about flexibility. It is true that some styles of yoga focus more on static stretching than on offering balanced and varied movement practices. This book is one of many emerging in the field to contribute to a dialogue on how we can create a more sustainable approach to yoga practice that supports the overall health and longevity of all the body's systems.

What is the difference between mobility and flexibility, you might ask? Flexibility is more about the length of a muscle. It can be one component of mobility, meaning that the length of a muscle might affect the ability of a joint to move through a specific range of motion. Other things that can affect mobility include some of what we discussed in chapter 5: joint structure, ligament laxity or tightness, past or present injuries, and psychology. Of course, the added component that we want you to consider is the nervous system—developing that focused ability to apply motor (neural) control to differentiated joint actions in a variety of positions. Think of mobility as an equation for how a balanced joint moves—a sweet combination of flexibility, motor control, and stability. Instead of working on flexibility for flexibility's sake, we are asking that you put flexibility into the larger context of how it affects other aspects of your movement practices and overall functioning. While you're learning, make sure that the gains you make in flexibility are examined in relationship to your ability to actually control the range of motion in a particular joint.

Beyond the poses, you can relate the intention of mobility to aspects of your life by considering your emotional mobility: How easily are you moved? Can you experience a range of emotions while staying connected to yourself and others? How about your thoughts? Is your mental state agile and adaptable? Can you navigate the different aspects of your life with a sense of solid presence and free thinking?

Strength

The options in this category focus on joint stability, core awakening, postural control, relaxing antagonist muscles, and recruiting stabilizer muscles. Here we introduce experiences that use the wall or props to help awaken muscle activity, add weight, or increase the number of repetitions. Some options will require static strength and others will focus on strength through movement.

Beyond the poses, you can relate the category of strength to daily life by doing what is necessary to stay on track to meet your goals, even when it is difficult or challenges other people's needs and expectations for you. Notice your ability to maintain emotional balance in intense situations or express your thoughts even when they might not be in line with popular thinking. These and other subtle adaptations require a strong sense of self.

Balance

This category focuses on the ability to stay upright in both static and dynamic positions. The options explore signals to the brain sent by the joints, eyes, and inner ear. We will often do this by introducing asymmetrical and cross-body movement patterns that will challenge the body's sensory systems. As you explore this category, remember that balance is more than just standing on one foot! It is something that can happen on two feet and in orientations other than standing.

Beyond the poses, a balanced lifestyle requires practice, especially in busy, modern times. You can relate the intention of balance to how you schedule work, rest, and leisure time. You may notice certain requirements for keeping your energy levels balanced, where you are neither overly active and on the edge of burnout, nor overly sedentary, slothful, or listless. A balanced mind or emotional state expresses clarity, interest, and variability. It also achieves harmony between accepting internal and external circumstances and taking action to change what needs changing.

Recovery

The options in this category focus on more passive or relaxed variations of the poses and breathing explorations. They are intended to help the body relax and reduce the nervous system's response to stimulus. This is accomplished through the use of props to support the body and engender release. As you explore this section, think of these variations as choices to help you slow down and let go. You can use them to help the body recover from vigorous activity, to prepare the body and mind for sleep, to offer support during times of illness, or to help quiet the mind during times of stress.

Beyond the poses, you can relate the intention of recovery to other aspects of your life by considering the amount of time you take between tasks or the space you give yourself to reflect on and assimilate daily emotions and experiences. How often do you give yourself time for rest in general? Remember that rest can be different from sleep; sleep is just one component of rest, albeit an important one. You may especially notice a subtle, quiet connection with yourself while exploring periods of recovery.

Joint Differentiation

A skillful, personalized yoga therapy program requires practitioners to be aware of how their joints move. This next section offers positional micro-sequences intended to bring awareness to basic joint movements. Engaging with the sequences mindfully should help to increase proprioception and general positional joint awareness during more complicated poses or activities. Start by doing them slowly and with a focus on detail. As you break them down, you will notice that they relate to a lot of the activities that you do in daily life.

The sequences function as awareness-building practices that pair nicely with other orientations such as seated, table, or standing. Think of the sequences as a foundation from which you can build a clearer understanding of your options in your pose experiences. Once you are familiar with the joint differentiations, you can use them as a gentle warm-up or cool-down practice or even practice them by themselves at the end of a stressful day to encourage downregulation of the nervous system through gentle movement.

From a big-picture perspective, the sequences offer a framework from which you can become more aware of how your nervous system, joints, muscles, and fascia come together to function. When you slow the explorations and pay attention to how you are doing them (**identification**), you will open up to new movement options in practice (**differentiation**) and in your daily life and activities (**integration**). This means paying attention to the obvious sensations at first, and over time becoming more sensitive to the not-so-obvious sensations as your yoga therapy practice evolves.

In previous chapters, we talked about the importance of slow movement for enhanced learning. Slowing down, paying attention to, and sensing the subtle aspects of how the joints move can be more difficult than it sounds, especially when the physical body mirrors the mental or emotional aspects of your experience. Many people we encounter are challenged in some way by slowing down and paying attention. This includes novices as well as experienced yoga practitioners, who may have developed a habit of overriding or sublimating some of the more subtle joint feedback in their practice instead of being present with it. It's normal to resist new levels of awareness and the potential ensuing change. Again, be patient with yourself as you try to choose the appropriate level of challenge for your nervous system so that even during times of effort, you experience a sense of curiosity, ease, and receptivity as you explore.

The movement explorations in this section offer the potential for awareness of healthy ranges of motion in the major joints of the body. The first few sequences for the upper and lower body are done lying down. There is a purpose for this. When you lie down, you don't have to use your habitual postural muscles to hold you up, so it is easier to move in new, non-habitual ways. Too much of the nervous system is already engaged when you are standing, and it is then more difficult to let the nervous system recalibrate or introduce new movements without layering on an already present layer.

Lying down also offers an effective pre- and post-exploration check-in mechanism if you start and end each sequence in a comparatively reclined position (knees bent or legs straight) to notice the impact of the practices on how you perceive yourself lying on the ground. The positional check-in offers the potential for greater insight into the small changes that happen in the body and mind during each set of movements.

Once you have differentiated the joints in a reclined position, you can differentiate the same movement patterns in other, more physically demanding positions. For example, you can also perform the neck series from standing, and while you might use the same combination of muscles, the way that you experience them lying down will be different from the way that you experience them standing up.

Reclined Neck Series

As you explore the reclined neck series, pay attention to the changing points of contact of the back of the head on the floor during the movements. You can perform the entire series from a partially reclined position with the knees bent and feet on the floor or fully reclined with the legs straight on the floor.

Flexion and extension: Inhale to move the chin away from the chest and toward the ceiling (a). Exhale to bring the chin back down toward the chest (b). Repeat 5 to 10 times.

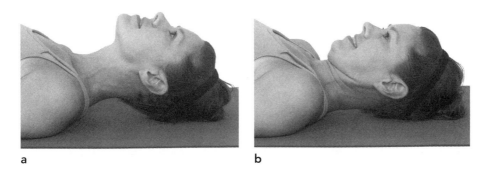

a   b

Rotation: Inhale to turn the neck to the left. Exhale to bring the head back to center. Inhale to turn to the right. Exhale to come back to center. Repeat 5 to 10 times.

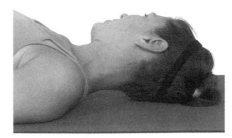

Lateral flexion: Inhale to lower the right ear toward the right shoulder. Exhale to return the head to center. Inhale to lower the left ear toward the left shoulder. Exhale to return to center. Repeat 5 to 10 times.

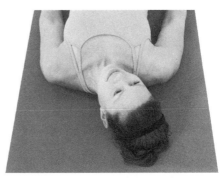

Small circles: Draw small clockwise circles in the air with the nose. Pay attention to the changing points of contact between the back of the head and the floor. Repeat 5 to 10 times and then circle in the opposite direction.

Figure 8: Draw small figure 8s in the air with the nose. Pay attention to the changing points of contact between the back of the head and the floor. Repeat 5 to 10 times and then move in the opposite direction.

Reclined Shoulder Series

You can perform this series from a reclined position with the knees bent and feet on the floor or reclined with the legs straight out. As you explore the movements, pay attention to the spine. What is it like to allow the spine to move along with the shoulders compared to keeping the spine still while the shoulders move?

Flexion and extension: Start with the arms active by the sides of the body, a few inches off of the ground with the palms facing the floor (a). Inhale to lift both arms skyward, eventually raising them until they are beside the ears (b). Exhale to lower the arms back down by the sides of the body. Repeat 5 to 10 times.

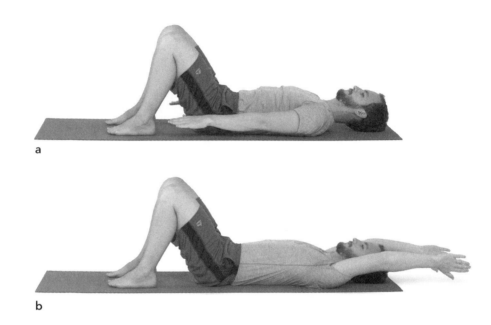

Internal and external rotation: Bring the arms out to the sides at shoulder height with the elbows bent at 90 degrees, and the forearms and palms facing the wall in front of you (a). With an inhalation, roll through the upper-arm bones to bring the forearms down toward the floor (b). Keep the upper arms straight out from the shoulders and the elbows bent at 90 degrees throughout the movement. Exhale to return to the starting position. Roll through the upper-arm bones to bring the hands towards the ears and the forearms toward the ceiling (c). Repeat 5 to 10 times.

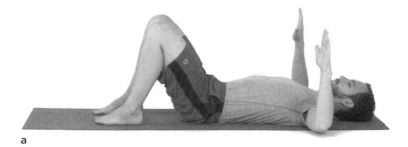

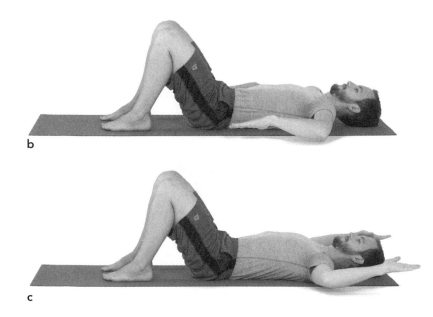

b

c

Protraction and retraction: Reach arms straight toward the ceiling, shoulder-width apart, and palms facing each other. Inhale and reach toward the ceiling, spreading the shoulder blades apart *(a)*. Exhale as the shoulder blades slide back toward the floor and each other *(b)*. Repeat 5 to 10 times.

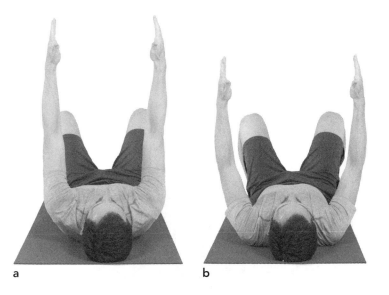

a   b

Angel arms: Begin with arms beside the body, and a few inches off of the floor with the palms towards the ground. Roll the shoulders open and palms towards the sky as you sweep the arms out to the sides and then up by the ears. Keep the arms straight as you reach toward the ceiling and bring them back down to the sides of the body.

Repeat 5 to 10 times and then reverse the movement by starting with the arms by the ears with the palms up, sweeping them out to the sides as you roll the shoulders closed. Turn the palms back toward the ground, and return the arms back to the sides of body.

Pelvis Series

Even though the focus of this series is on moving the pelvis, the reclined version asks that you also pay attention to the relationship between the entire spine and the floor as you move. After you get a sense of doing the pelvic movements from a reclined position with the knees bent and feet on the mat, you can also try them with the legs straight or the soles of the feet together and the knees opened out to the sides. See how the different hip positions change your experience.

Posterior and anterior tilt: Inhale to slowly roll the front of the pelvis toward the feet (anterior tilt), creating space between the low back and the floor *(a)*. Exhale to roll the front of the pelvis toward the head (posterior tilt), connecting the low back to the floor *(b)*. Repeat 5 to 10 times going forward and backward.

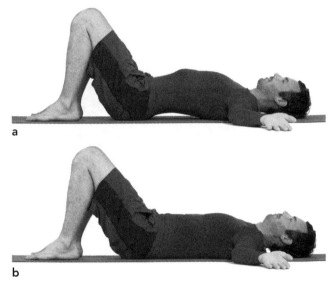

Side to side: Exhale to shift weight into the right side of the pelvis as the left side lifts slightly away from the ground. Inhale back to center. Exhale to shift weight to the left side of the pelvis, allowing the right side to slightly lift. Repeat 5 to 10 times, moving from side to side.

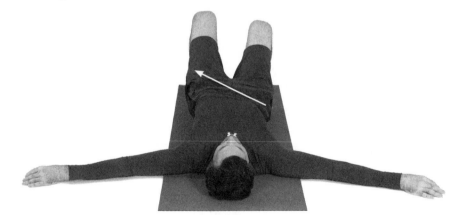

Circular: Visualize a circle under your low back, the base of the circle at the tip of the sacrum and the top of the circle under the navel. Move the pelvis forward, backward, and sideways to trace the imaginary circle. Repeat 5 to 10 times, and then trace the circle in the opposite direction.

Now play with making your circle smaller or larger, noticing how that changes the movement for you. Switch the focus to the front of the body by visualizing that you are drawing a circle on the ceiling with a flashlight in your navel. How does the movement or awareness change when you focus on the front instead of the back of the body?

Spine Series

This series focuses on spinal articulation from a reclined, kneeling, and belly-down position. Perform the movements slowly while visualizing each vertebra as a pearl on a string, each pearl moving when it is ready. As you explore this series, see whether you can focus on creating a fluid quality of movement in the spine as you come into and out of the shapes.

Bridge: Start in a reclined position with the knees bent, feet on the mat, arms by the sides of the body, and palms down and pressing lightly into the floor. Bring the feet hip-width apart under the knees.

Inhale to roll the front of the pelvis toward the head and pick it up off of the ground. Continue the movement into the midspine, allowing each vertebra to lift off the ground, one after the other. Stop the articulation when the elevated pelvis is in line with the thighbones.

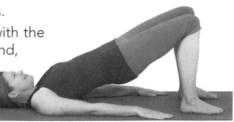

Exhale to reverse the movement, starting with the midspine back down to the ground. As you land, let the front of the pelvis roll toward the feet and create a small space between the low back and the floor. Repeat 5 to 10 times.

Cat–cow: Position yourself on all fours with hands under the shoulders and knees under the hips. Keep space between the knees.

Exhale to roll the pelvis under the body, continuing the movement into the midspine and neck, slowly articulating into roundness. Press the hands into the floor to help spread the shoulder blades apart at the top of the movement (a).

Inhale to reverse the articulation, slowly articulating the pelvis, midspine and head in the opposite direction into a backbend (b). Repeat 5 to 10 times.

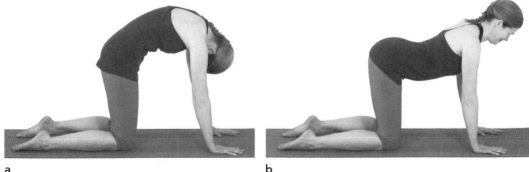

a   b

Cobra articulation: Start in a belly-down position with the legs straight behind the body. Bend the elbows and bring them in line with the torso, lightly pressing the palms into the mat with the fingertips in line with the shoulders.

Inhale to lift the breastbone, slowly peeling the front of the body off of the ground, keeping the neck in line with the rest of the spine.

Exhale to slowly articulate the front of the body back down to the mat. Repeat 5 to 10 times.

Reclined Foot, Leg, and Hip Series

This series focuses on pairing different ankle and hip movements with core stability. As you explore, keep equal weight in the pelvis (both buttocks on the ground), activating the core, and maintaining pelvic stability as you move through the hip joint. The instructions offer the feedback of the yoga strap, but the series can also be done hands free. Without the support of the strap, more focus and core stability is required. You can explore the series step by step, alternating from leg to leg in each exercise or by doing the entire series on one leg and then again on the other.

Plantarflexion and dorsiflexion: Start in a reclined position with both knees bent and both feet on the mat.

Bring the left knee in toward the chest and place a yoga strap across the ball of the left foot, holding an end in each hand. Draw the strap taut as you raise the left leg toward the ceiling. Keep the shoulders relaxed and supported by the mat.

Articulate through the ankle as you point the foot away from the shin (plantarflexion) into the light resistance of the strap, (a) and bring the foot toward the shin (dorsiflexion) (b) with the assistance of the strap. Repeat 5 to 10 times.

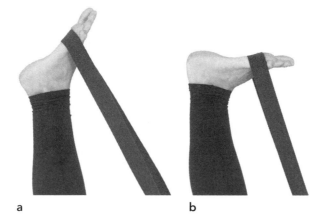

a   b

Inversion and eversion: Move the strap down to the arch of the foot. Roll the ankle sideways, bringing the outside of the foot toward the outer edge of the right leg as the inside of the foot comes away from the inside of the leg (eversion) (a).

Return to center and bring the inside edge of the foot toward the inner leg line and the outside of the foot away from the outside of the leg (inversion) (b). Repeat 5 to 10 times, moving from side to side.

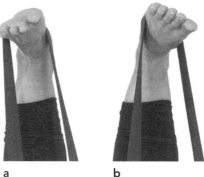

a   b

Ankle circles: Place the strap on the ball of the foot, continuing to pull it lightly taut. Circle the ankle into the feedback of the strap, exploring how the pointing, flexing, and side-to-side action come together to create the feeling of circling. Repeat 5 to 10 times, then move the circle in the opposite direction.

Hip circles: Place the strap on the arch of the foot, continuing to pull it lightly taut. Focus on where the thighbone connects to the pelvis. Use the strap to guide a small circular hip action, maintaining equal weight in the pelvis as you move. Repeat 5 to 10 times, and then circle in the opposite direction.

Leg-stretch variation 1: Bend the left knee and bring it toward the chest (a). Keep the strap on the arch of the foot, continuing to pull it lightly taut as you straighten the knee to raise the foot toward the ceiling. Stop straightening the knee when you start to feel the hamstring stretch in the back of the leg (b). Pause here for a few breaths without straightening the knee any more or drawing the leg any closer toward you.

After a few breaths, play with the degree of bend in the knee and with how close you draw the leg to the torso, adjusting as needed for your body. Hold for 1 to 2 minutes. Repeat with the other leg.

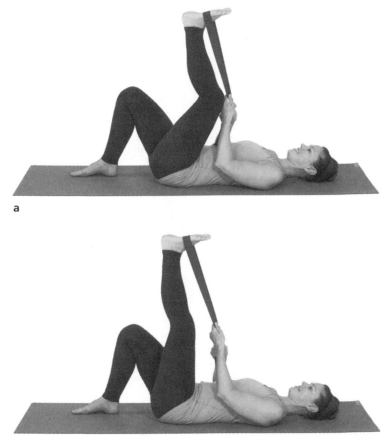

a

b

Leg-stretch variation 2: Start in leg-stretch variation 1 with the left leg skyward. Open the leg out to the left, keeping equal weight in the pelvis.

Pull the strap taut to support the weight of the leg against gravity and draw the leg slightly up and in toward the ear.

For extra support, hold the strap in the right hand and use the left hand to help hold up the leg. Hold for 1 to 2 minutes. Repeat with the other leg.

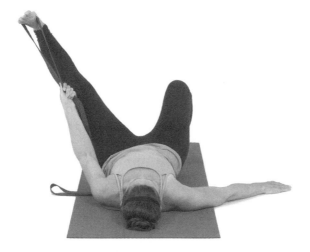

Leg-stretch variation 3: Start in leg-stretch variation 1 with the left leg skyward. Keep equal weight in the pelvis as you draw the left leg across the midline of the body. Pull the strap taut to help support the weight of the leg. Hold for 1 to 2 minutes. Repeat with the other leg.

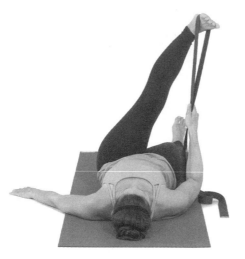

Now that you have differentiated your joint movements, continue preparing for the following chapter by further exploring the core.

Dead Bug Series

This short core-awakening series pairs pelvic stability with hip and shoulder mobility. Start the explorations with the knees bent at 90 degrees. Once you are able to maintain pelvic stability in the movements with the legs bent, you can make this series more challenging by straightening the legs. Only increase the challenge if you can maintain equal weight in the pelvis and core activation in the first position.

Static: Start in a reclined position with the knees bent and feet on the mat. Reach the arms toward the ceiling. Pick one foot off the floor at a time. Align the thighbones over the pelvis and line up the shins with the knees. Hold for 30 to 60 seconds.

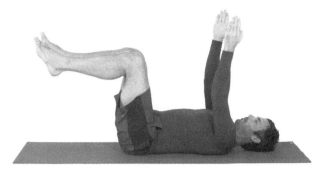

Tip: Flowing dead bug variations can also be done with the knees bent, as pictured for the static variation or with the legs long as seen.

Flowing variation 1: Start in the basic position. Inhale to bring the left leg down toward the floor without touching it and the right arm up toward right ear. Exhale to bring the arm and leg back into the starting position. Repeat, alternating from side to side 5 to 10 times.

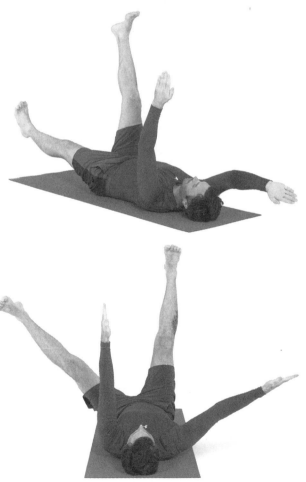

Flowing variation 2: Start in the basic position. Inhale to bring the right arm out to the right side and left leg out to the left side. Keep the abdomen engaged and extend only as far out and down as you can while maintaining equal weight in the pelvis. Exhale to bring the arm and leg back to the starting position. Repeat, moving from side to side 5 to 10 times.

Flowing variation 3: From the basic position, circle the right arm and the left hip at the same time, drawing circles on the ceiling, focusing on keeping the movement small and in the shoulder and hip sockets. Repeat 5 to 10 times, moving the opposite arm and leg at the same time, and then move in the opposite direction. Next move the arm and the leg in opposite directions (i.e., arm circles to the right and leg circles to the left). Repeat on the opposite partnered sides.

EXPLORATION
Spine in Active Neutral

This exploration layers in the elements of previously highlighted concepts to create a new concept called active neutral. The active-neutral cue is woven into many of the movement instructions in coming chapters, so we will explore it here by itself before you apply it to the yoga pose variations.

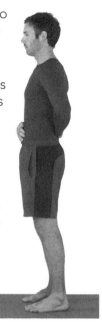

1 Start by standing with the feet hip-width apart and the arms at the sides of the body. Bring a sense of downward energy into the arms and fingers as you reach towards the floor. Ground yourself equally onto all three points—base of big toe, base of little toe, center of heel—of each foot.

2 Play with tucking and untucking your pelvis to feel the curve of the low back. Can you do this without placing the spine in an overly arched (backbend) or overly flexed (forward bend) position? Put one hand on the front of the abdomen and the other on the low back. Can you find equal tension in both hands? This is an indicator that you have found neutral. Visualize the natural curves of the spine being supported by the core.

3 Inhale into your abdomen, purposefully puffing out the lower belly as you do so. Retain your breath and draw everything that you have just puffed out back toward the spine into a light abdominal brace. Can you do this without going into a backbend or forward bend? Review abdominal bracing in chapter 7 if needed.

4 Repeat the breathing and light bracing a few times, holding the breath to get a sense of the stabilizing contraction and changes of intraabdominal pressure you are creating. Continue to visualize the natural curves of the spine being supported by the abdominal brace.

5 Once you sense how to do this, try to do the same thing without holding the breath. Can you breathe into the rib cage and abdomen as you maintain a light abdominal brace?

6 Explore different levels of the abdominal brace as you continue to breathe into your abdomen and rib cage. Try it at 25, 50, 75, and 100 percent. Which level allows you to find yourself upright, strong, and connected to your core, supporting the natural curves of the spine without being too rigid in your support or too soft and without support? How does your body balance effort and relaxation while maintaining active neutral in a standing position?

Now that you have explored personal intentions for practice, deconstructed potential physical intentions for yoga poses, differentiated joint movements, and explored the concept of active neutral, you are well prepared to move on to the yoga asana explorations in the next chapters. Get ready to continue your journey of identification, differentiation, and integration in yoga pose practice!

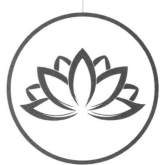

nine
Spinal Movement Poses

This chapter applies the principles of identification, differentiation, and integration to common categories of yoga poses. We will start with four categories that relate to the movements of the spine: forward fold, backbend, side bend, and twist. The idea is that yoga therapy practitioners need to differentiate how their spines move before they explore more complex categories of poses. What you learn from the first four categories is important in itself, and it becomes even more important when you relate it to making differentiated choices in the final four categories of pose variations: core, standing, balance, and hips. Many variations in those categories include options for exploring differentiated spinal movements within the context of a particular pose.

As you explore this chapter, try to approach each pose with a curious attitude. Stay away from value judgments (such as good or bad) if you can. If your first reaction is a strong like or dislike, do your best to move beyond that surface reaction and uncover what it really means in terms of your needs and potential learning. In other words, be curious about—rather than simply believing—your initial responses. Movements that you might like or that feel good to you may be ones that solidify present habits. See whether you can go further than like or dislike to look at *how* you are doing something and what options you have for doing it differently.

Overview of the Identification Process

The **identification** process uses the same structure for each pose. This means we expect you to inquire into the pose that you are doing from both a top-down (thinking, external focus, alignment, body position) and bottom-up (internal sensation, intuitive movement, feeling) perspective. To reduce redundancies, we do not repeat the identification inquiry at the beginning of each pose. Please remember to use it! Revisit the identification process after you have completed the variations. This offers an opportunity to gain a greater understanding of your movement patterns that will inform the integration process.

Let's walk through what the identification process might look like for each pose.

Top Down

- Perform the pose. Pay attention to the physical choices that you make, the "how" of the movements. Do it a few more times if necessary to start discerning the external habits of this particular pose.
- From what location do you initiate the movement to come into the shape? To come back out?
- What do you physically feel in your body? Where do you feel it?
- How do you sense your skeletal alignment in the pose? Where are your feet, pelvis, spine, shoulders, and head in relationship to each other?
- How mobile do you feel? Where do you feel relaxation or freedom in the body?
- How stable are you? Where do you feel muscular engagement?
- How aware are you of your pelvis and core while entering, holding, and exiting the pose?
- How do you use your breath while entering, holding, and exiting the pose? How do you breathe during an extended hold versus a shorter hold?
- Make notes of what you noticed and learned.

Bottom Up

- Perform the pose. Pay attention to how you feel coming into and out of it. Repeat as needed to discern the internal habits of this pose.
- What is your attitude toward the pose? Where does that come from? Is it an attitude that you brought to the pose, or did the pose create the attitude?
- What is your emotional reaction to the pose? Is it just one emotion or does it change over time?
- What does this pose reveal to you about your quality of mind? For example, are you focused, restless, calm, agitated, or distracted? Does holding the pose for a while change your quality of mind?
- What thoughts, sounds, vocalizations, visuals, or colors emerge during the pose?
- Where do you feel energy moving or awakening in the pose? Where does the energy feel stuck or dull?
- If you take a pause from your conditioned reactions or expectations about the pose, what awareness is possible?
- Make note of what you noticed.

Overview of the Differentiation Process

The **differentiation** process will often have similarities in each category or pose. Whenever they are different or more specific to the category or pose we are exploring, they will be offered in the beginning of that section via an exploration exercise. These general differentiations can be applied to most poses.

Differentiate the Breath

- ○ Exhale into a pose. Inhale to come out. Now try the reverse.
- ○ Experiment with focusing the breath in either the rib cage or the lower back and abdomen rather than connecting the two.
- ○ Try prolonging the inhalation and exhalation instead of using a more natural and easy breathing rhythm.
- ○ Try a full cycle of breath during the different phases of the pose. In other words, take a full inhale and exhale as you enter, another inhale and exhale as you hold, and another inhale and exhale as you exit.
- ○ Try using the breathing rhythm to slow or speed the entering, holding, and exiting of the pose.

Differentiate and Link Parts to the Whole

- ○ How do you use your feet and legs in different variations? How wide or narrow is your base? What position is your pelvis in? How does that relate to the position of your spine and hips?
- ○ How do you use your shoulders, arms, and hands in different variations? What position are your shoulders in?
- ○ How do you use your jaw, face, or eyes?
- ○ How does the experience change when you focus on the front of the body rather than the back of the body? What about if you focus on the relationship between the front and back of the body?
- ○ How much effort are you using? Where is effort necessary or helpful? Where is relaxation necessary or helpful? What is the balance required between effort and relaxation?

Differentiate a Variety of Intentions

- ○ **Energetic:** Focus on energy moving. Where does it feel free flowing? Where does it feel stuck? How do physical choices move or change the energetic awareness?
- ○ **Emotional:** Focus on the emotions that the pose elicits for you. Notice whether they change during the pose.
- ○ **Mental:** Focus on harnessing inward attention, calmness, and a meditative mindset.
- ○ **Spiritual:** Focus on qualities such as acceptance, surrender, or freedom.

Overview of the Integration Process

The **integration** process always asks that you come back to the identification process to see what you have learned and then asks that you apply your learning to the activities that you enjoy. Even though we don't remind you after each category or pose variation, remember that it is up to you to acknowledge the learning that happened through the pose explorations so that you can integrate it into your daily life.

Integration Points of Focus

- Come back to the identification process. Do you have a better idea of your options for and experiences of this particular pose or category of poses? Do you know what combinations of the top-down or bottom-up approach might work for your intentions?

- Pay attention to all the activities in your life to which that category of movement or pose applies. Where is it helpful? Where is it not? How can the awareness that you have gained from your explorations help you make more integrated choices in daily activities?

You will notice as you apply the concepts of identification, differentiation, and integration that this chapter offers a lot of work on differentiation. As you play with differentiating, you may notice that too much differentiation can become confusing or discouraging. Not enough differentiation and your movements may stay or become habitual. Try to strike a balance between challenging and overwhelming yourself. Often, you will have to walk a fine line to discover an appropriate equilibrium for your nervous system.

While we would love to offer you every variation of every yoga pose possible, we are limited by the nature of the written format. Within that context, we do our best to offer examples that you can use to build a foundation from which you can continue to explore. When you have differentiated all of the poses that we have to offer, we hope you will use this framework to engage with other variations, poses, and movements that might be outside of the scope of this book, as well as creating some unique variations of your own!

Forward Fold

Whether you are an experienced yoga practitioner or a newbie, spinal flexion is a familiar movement pattern. We spend the first nine months of our lives in the womb in flexion, and return to flexion as we age. Birth to death, flexion is one of the primary movement patterns of human life.

Modern times have caged us in cars, chairs, desks, and in front of electronics. Many of us are stuck in spinal flexion because of the amount of sitting required for work and other common daily activities. This results in lots of people holding their thoracic and cervical spines in a C-curve, with their heads forward, often coupled with tucked or posteriorly tilted pelvises. When a person is stuck in flexion all day, it becomes a postural habit that can wreak havoc on all the systems of the body.

Mindfulness is required to identify how much spinal flexion you experience during daily life. Once you get a sense of that, you can start to differentiate positions that give you options instead of staying in one position all day. If you can't change your seated position while you work, try to get up and move as much as possible. If you are stuck in a chair, you could roll out your feet under the desk (see the tennis ball exploration in chapter 7) or work on opening the front of the body throughout the course of the day. To help balance out excessive spinal flexion, you could also adapt the movements of the spine outlined in this chapter and do them at your desk. Whatever you can do to add variety of movement within the confines of your work environment will be helpful.

Recently the yoga community has debated whether or not spinal flexion is beneficial, especially in yoga classes for the general public. Some teachers have argued for taking spinal flexion off the menu entirely and others for modifying it to a degree that greatly restricts the movement. We tend to fall into the middle ground and are of the opinion that if the spine was not meant to flex, it wouldn't. If your body is overly taxed by forward folds in an unhelpful way, we suggest reducing the amount of forward folding along with exploring the forward-folding differentiations in this section to get a better sense of how much and which variations are helpful and which are not.

If you are unsure about how far to go or how hard to try in these pose variations, less can be more. It isn't about touching your toes, getting your head to your knees, or even being able to do the most difficult variations. It's about discerning your habits and becoming more responsive to them. It's about introducing options for different experiences in the same pose while continuing to identify and work intelligently with limitations that might come up. Think of doing a well-rounded and moderate yoga therapy practice as preventive care for your spine, attempting to move it in all the directions it can move throughout the course of each day.

As you become more aware of your postural habits, you will be able to make more conscious choices about how you hold yourself in the world. As you will see, many of the spinal movements we offer in this chapter can be related to the activities of daily life. During the explorations in this chapter, take notes on your experiences. This will allow you to track your growing awareness over time and better understand how your yoga therapy practices are evolving. Happy forward folding!

EXPLORATION
Forward Fold

❶ Start standing with the feet hip-width apart, arms by the sides, and the spine in active neutral. Bend the knees slightly. Keep the head, shoulders, pelvis, and spine in one line, and engage some core support as you focus on folding forward from the hip creases.

❷ Walk the hands down onto the thighs, shins, or blocks. Knees can stay bent in order to maintain a small lumbar curve. Only lower as far as you can while maintaining active neutral in the spine.

❸ Now reverse the order of the movement, keeping the spine in active neutral as you hinge from the hips to return to standing.

❹ Start in standing again. Initiate the folding-forward movement from the head and upper spine, rounding toward the ground. Keep the knees bent as you continue to roll, vertebra by vertebra, through the spine down toward the floor.

❺ Reverse and slowly roll back up to standing, initiating with the pelvis curling under into a posterior tilt. Try to tap into core support while you articulate back up.

❻ Start in standing again. Keep the head, neck, and spine in one line as you fold forward from the hip creases. At the end of the hip flexion, slowly let the upper spine round toward the floor and legs. Knees can be slightly bent in order to accommodate any restriction that you might come across in the pelvis or hamstrings.

❼ Reverse the order of the movement to return to standing, moving from roundness into active neutral before hinging from the hips to come up.

❽ Now that you have differentiated these aspects of forward fold (focus on the spine versus the hips versus pairing both together) can you sense how the different intentions for initiating the forward fold change your experience?

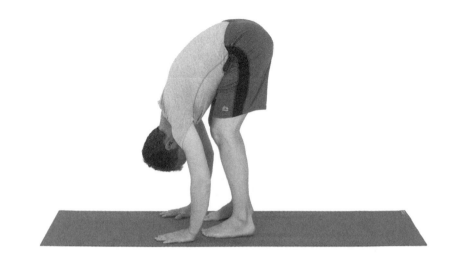

1. Start by standing with the feet hip-width apart, arms active and straight along the sides of the body and the spine in active neutral. Slightly bend the knees and tuck or untuck the pelvis to find an appropriate lumbar curve.

2. Hinge forward from the hips, using a light abdominal brace in tandem with your breath to keep the spine in active neutral on the way down. Review the breathing with abdominal bracing exercise in chapter 7 if needed.

3. Bring hands to the thighs, shins, or floor as you round the spine. Play with how much or how little bend in the knees your body needs.

4. Hold 30 to 90 seconds.

TIP: Before coming into a forward fold, some people need to tuck (posteriorly tilt) the pelvis, others need to untuck (anteriorly tilt) the pelvis to find the lumbar curve appropriate for their body. Revisit the reclined pelvis series in chapter 8 if you need to review this foundational movement pattern.

Basic Options

Partial entry: From the basic position, keep the hands or forearms on the thighs and use a deeper knee bend (a).

Legs form narrow base: Bring the feet and legs together (b).

Legs form wide angle: Stand with the legs 2 to 3 feet (61-91 cm) apart. The spine can be in active neutral or rounded, with or without blocks (c).

Hands on blocks: At the bottom of the movement, put hands on blocks on the medium (long and narrow) or high (tall and perpendicular to the floor) setting lined up on the floor (d).

Arms behind the body: At the bottom of the movement, reach the arms behind the body, palms facing each other (e). Clasp the hands or grasp a yoga strap in each hand. Allow the arms to move toward the head once you have folded forward (f).

Arms sideways during entry and exit: Bring the arms out to the sides of the body, active at shoulder height.

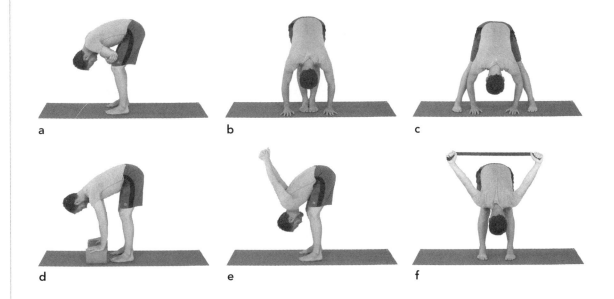

a   b   c

d   e   f

Mobility Options

Upper-body focus at the wall: Position the buttocks against the wall. The legs are in front of you and knees slightly bent.

Let the lower spine come into contact with the wall as you gently drop the chin to the chest while rounding the upper and middle spine and neck. Allow the arms to hang as you give the upper body over to the pull of gravity *(a)*.

Asymmetrical: Before folding forward from a standing position, place the left foot on a block. Line up the toes of both feet next to each other. The feet are hip-width apart. Bend the left knee and level the pelvis. Remain standing as you practice straightening and bending the knee, allowing the left hip to elevate as you keep the right foot on the ground. This is the action that will be required after folding forward.

Fold forward from the hip creases. Round the spine (flexion), with the hands on blocks or the floor. Start to straighten the knee, letting the hip and buttock elevate toward the ceiling *(b)*. Pay attention to the sensations in the left hamstrings and the outer edge of the left hip. Play with how much or little bend you need to keep in the knee. Sense your natural end ranges and honor them without forcing the stretch.

Hold for 30 to 90 seconds. Bend the left knee, level the pelvis, and bring the spine back to active neutral before hip hinging back to standing.

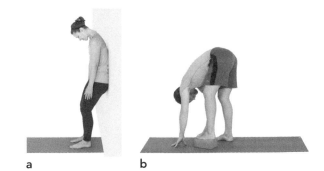

a   b

Strength Options

These strengthening variations can build core awareness. Only straighten the knees if you can maintain active neutral in the spine in tandem with a light abdominal brace.

At the wall: Using the same instructions as for the basic standing forward fold, face a wall. Walk your hands down the wall, bring the arms in line with the shoulder as you press your palms into the wall and create an L-shape with your body. Bend the knees as much as needed to keep the spine in active neutral (pelvis, spine, neck, and head in one line). Try to find and maintain the stability of the shoulder blades without flaring the ribs or going into a backbend (a). Once you have a sense of that activity, disconnect one hand from the wall and play with taking the arm back toward the leg and out at shoulder height.

Hands-free variation 1: From the L-shape at the wall, slowly remove the hands from the wall and play with putting the shoulders and arms in different positions. Start with the arms straight and active at the sides, palms facing the floor (b).

Hands-free variation 2: Arms are straight and active at shoulder height, palms facing the floor (c).

Hands-free variation 3: Arms are straight and next to the ears with the palms facing each other. Hands are no longer touching the wall, so you may need to back away from the wall a bit for this variation (d).

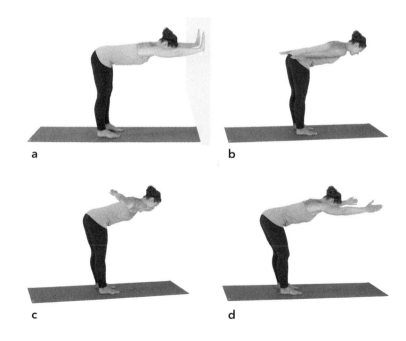

a

b

c

d

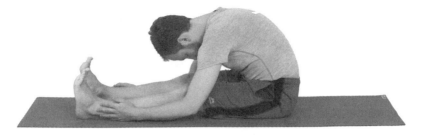

1 Start in a seated position with the legs straight in front of you. If needed, elevate the pelvis on a blanket or bolster in order to find an appropriate lumbar curve.

2 Exhale to hinge from the hips and lower the torso toward the thighs. When you feel the unforced end range of the hip hinge, allow the spine to round toward the legs. The feet can be pointed or flexed.

3 Hands rest on the shins, thighs, or ground next to the legs. If you can reach the feet naturally, hold there. Try not to use your hands to pull yourself farther into the fold. Sense your natural end ranges and honor them without forcing the stretch.

4 Hold 30 to 90 seconds.

Basic Options

Bent knees: You can bend the knees deeply with the feet on the ground, or bend them slightly and tuck a rolled blanket under them. With a deep knee bend, the torso can rest on the thighs. Hands can rest on the floor or gently hug the shins (a).

Butterfly: Bring the soles of the feet together and the knees out to the side. Heels can be close to the groin or a little farther away (b).

Wide angle: Open the legs so that feet are 2 to 3 feet (61-91 cm) apart (c).

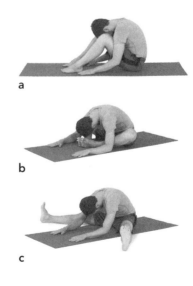

a

b

c

Mobility Option

Articulating forward fold: Start either upright with both knees bent in front of the torso and feet on the floor, or seated in a crossed-legged position with the arms out to the sides of the body. Exhale, hinge back from the hips *(a)*, and slowly articulate the mid- and upper-spine into a C-shape as you bend the elbows and touch your fingertips in front of the body (as if you were hugging a ball) *(b)*. Hold the shape for one breath cycle and reverse the movement back to neutral. Repeat 5 to 10 times.

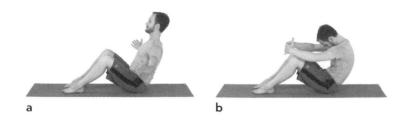

a   b

Recovery Options

For a more restorative experience, use props to give the body targeted support. This option works particularly well with the legs straight, at a wide angle, crossed, or in a butterfly position. Hold the supported variations for 1 to 3 minutes.

Bolstered: Drape the torso over a bolster or blanket stack. The bolster can be placed in between the legs or on top of them. Turn the head to rest on the bolster if you need to, and turn it to the other side midway through the pose *(a)*.

Chair: Place the upper body and arms on the seat of a chair. The forehead can rest on the edge of the chair if helpful *(b)*.

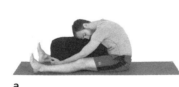 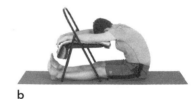

a   b

Backbend

When you become aware of just how much flexion is a part of your daily life, spinal extension comes along to give you new movement experiences to explore. Practically speaking, if you spend a lot of time in spinal flexion, spinal extension provides a counterbalance and awakening point for your movement practices.

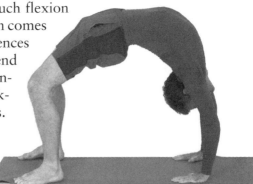

Wheel pose.

If you peel away the superficial layers of visual attraction of poses such as wheel or scorpion, you start to see that backbends ask you to move in a way that you are not accustomed to in daily life. For this reason, spinal extension might seem a little scary or unsafe at first. Backbends can trigger protective instincts in the body—and for good reason. On a primal level, you are wired to protect the front of the body from harm. To open the front of the body in extension requires showing your soft, vulnerable underbelly to the world. On the other side of that vulnerability and fear is the potential for the positives associated with opening the body. Healthy backbends can be an expression of power, openness, or focus that can invigorate, surprise, and delight you in practice and in life.

It may be a relief to hear that you don't have to strive for big, dramatic backbends like wheel or scorpion in order to become more "advanced" in

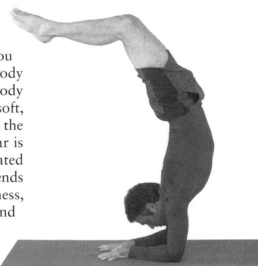

Scorpion pose.

your practice. Being advanced has nothing to do with mastering the extreme poses. In fact, you will not find any of what some might call advanced poses in this book. This does not mean that we think certain poses are bad, nor does it mean that we won't challenge you. It's just that our definition of advanced has more to do with awareness, options, and making conscious and integrated choices. As you may have already experienced, advanced challenges are found in giving the nervous system new movement puzzles to solve. For some of you, advanced awareness as we are defining it might actually ask you to regress in order to progress.

For all of these reasons and more, skillful backbends require a healthy sense of physical boundaries, mental focus, and a relaxed sense of curiosity. Think of it as a basic movement pattern that you can explore without having to strive too hard. At one point in your life, you were a baby on your belly, learning how to lift your head and engage your core. See whether you can use that image to help unlock playful focus and freedom for the following explorations. Happy backbending!

Backbend

1 Start by standing with the arms at the sides. Open the front of the body into a backbend. From where do you attempt to initiate the movement?

2 Now try holding the pelvis still as you initiate a backbend by lifting the breastbone skyward and articulating through the middle of the spine.

3 Can you find this movement through the midspine (thoracic) or is it somewhat restricted? If the movement is restricted in the midspine, where do you try to move from instead? The neck? The low back? The hips? Try again and see whether you can hold the lower body still and focus on the midspine movement.

4 Can you keep space and length in the back of the neck as you continue to focus on the movement in the thoracic spine? How does it change your experience?

5 Does bending back in this fashion keep you from going as far or deep as you are accustomed? Does the restriction help you focus your effort, set clearer boundaries, or move in a more aware or pain-free range?

6 Come in and out of the backbend a few more times while focusing on the relationship between your spine and shoulder blades. Can you sense how the shoulder blades slide back and toward each other as part of the natural sequence of thoracic-focused backbends? If not, can you allow your shoulder blades to participate in the movement?

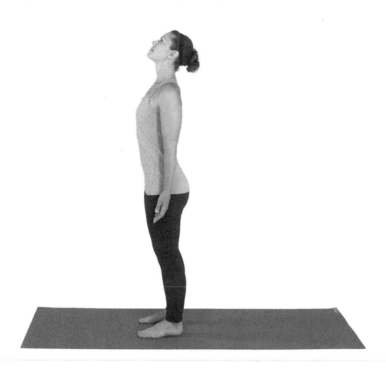

Standing Backbend

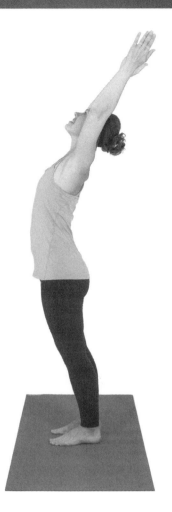

1. Start by standing with the feet hip-width apart, arms raised straight, next to the ears, and palms facing each other.

2. Ground yourself strongly into the triangle—base of the big toe, base of the pinky toe, center of the heel—on each foot. Tap into a light abdominal brace and activate the glutes.

3. Inhale to lift the chest skyward and create a small arch through the midback. The neck can stay neutral, or you can open the front of the throat slightly, maintaining space and length in the back of the neck.

4. Hold for 30 to 60 seconds.

Basic Options

Legs and stance variation 1: Change the base of the pose by bringing the legs together, insides of the feet and inner legs touching (a). You can also place a block or small exercise ball between the thighs to create more awareness of the inner leg and pelvic floor.

Legs and stance variation 2: Change the base of the pose by standing with the legs a little wider than shoulder-width apart. You can also do this variation with a strap around the upper thighs.

Arms: Position the arms behind the body with the palms facing each other or the wall behind you. You can do this variation with the hands free or holding a yoga strap taut between the hands (b).

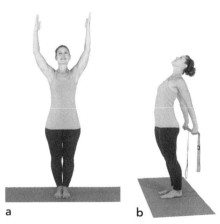

a   b

Balance Options

Split stance: Try any of the basic arm variations and place one foot in front of the other as if standing on a balance beam. Repeat on both sides, switching which leg is forward (a).

Single-leg variation 1: Start by standing with the feet hip-width apart. Bend the right knee and reach the right hand back to grab the top, inside, or outside of the right foot. Connect all three points of the standing foot to the ground.

Inhale to raise the left arm toward the ear with the palm facing the ceiling. Hinge forward from the left hip, lowering the torso slightly toward the floor. The right arm continues to reach behind the body as you press the right hand into the foot and the foot into the hand. Lift and open the chest. Remain with the torso leaning slightly toward the floor or continue to hinge from the hip to lower the torso to pelvis level.

Hold for 30 to 60 seconds and repeat on the other side (b).

Single-leg variation 2: Start by standing with the feet hip-width apart. Bend the left knee and gently lift it in toward the torso. Place the hands on the shin or use a strap to support the knee toward the chest.

Ground into the standing foot at all three points as you lift the chest and lean back slightly into a thoracic-focused backbend.

Hold for 30 to 60 seconds and repeat on the other side (c).

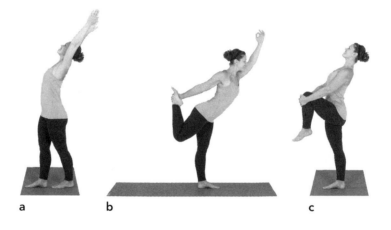

a b c

Recovery Option

Facing the wall: Stand facing the wall from approximately 1-2 feet (30-60 cm). Raise the arms long by the ears, and place the palms on the wall. Slightly bend both knees.

Hinge from the hips to bring the forehead and torso toward the wall, allowing the chest to expand and move slightly towards the wall as you arc into a mild backbend. Hold for 30 to 60 seconds and repeat on the other side.

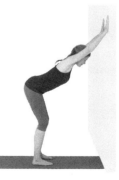

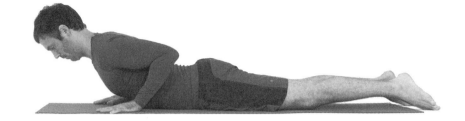

1. Start in a belly-down position, head and neck in line with the spine, legs straight out behind, and the tops of the feet on the floor. Elbows are bent at the sides of the body, palms are on the ground, and fingertips are lined up with the shoulders.

2. Gently press the hands into the ground to lift the upper body, initiating the backbend by raising and opening the chest and drawing the shoulder blades down and toward each other. Keep the neck neutral or open the throat slightly while maintaining space and length in the back of the neck.

3. Hold 30 to 60 seconds.

TIP: If your pelvis is uncomfortable against the floor in any of these positions, place a thin folded blanket under the bony hip points.

Basic Option

Partial entry: Cross the arms on the floor and stack one hand on top of the other. Prop the forehead on the hands. This may not seem like much of an exercise, but in this position, the body is in a very mild backbend that is supported by the floor.

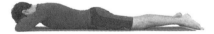

Mobility Option

Locust lifts variation 1: Start belly-down with the arms straight out in front on the floor. Inhale to lift the head, chest, and one arm and the opposite leg. Exhale to lower. Repeat lifting the other arm and leg. Perform side to side 5 to 10 times.

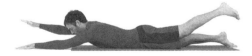

Strength Options

Locust lifts variation 2: This is similar to variation 1, but instead, raise both arms and both legs into a static hold, keeping all four limbs lifted while maintaining a light abdominal brace and focusing the breath into the rib cage. Hold for 15 to 60 seconds (a).

Cobra at the wall: Lie facedown on the floor with the legs straight, the feet flexed and pressing into the wall behind you. The arms are straight and positioned along each side of the body, the palms on the floor. As you lift the head and chest off the ground, contract the glutes, and press the palms into the floor. Hold for 15 to 60 seconds (b). This variation can also be done with the arms out to the sides at shoulder height or long by the ears.

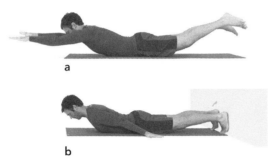

a

b

Recovery Option

TIP: The partial-entrance variation under basic variations also works well for recovery purposes.

Sphinx: Position the elbows under the shoulders and the forearms and palms on the ground. The head remains in line with the spine. The body can be a bit more relaxed in this variation. Try placing a bolster or blanket under the belly if it is helpful.

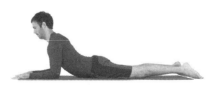

Reclined Backbend

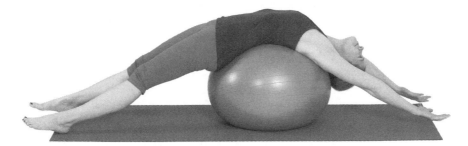

1. Start in a seated position on top of a medium-sized exercise ball. The spine is upright in active neutral, both knees are bent, and the feet are on the floor.

2. Walk the feet forward, slowly arching the length of the spine back onto the ball as you do so. The head can hang or the back of it can lightly touch the base of the ball.

3. Stay active through the core as you reach the arms above the head with the palms facing the ceiling. The shoulder blades contact the ball for support.

4. Knees can stay bent and the feet on the floor. Or you can walk the legs out with the heels on the floor.

5. Hold for 30 to 90 seconds.

Recovery Options

TIP: Use these leg positions for the recovery options: knees bent and feet on the mat, legs straight on the floor, or soles of the feet together with knees opened out to the sides.

Bolstered backbend: Start from a seated position with the knees bent and feet on the mat. Place a rectangular bolster or zed-folded blanket lengthwise behind the body. Tuck the end of it against the buttocks and low-back area.

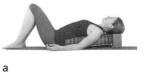

a

With an exhalation, lay the spine over the support of the bolster. The back of the head comes to rest on the bolster (or on a block tucked behind the bolster if the bolster is shorter than the torso). A small, rolled blanket or towel tucked into the curve of the back of the neck can also be helpful.

Take your time to settle into the support of the pose and adjust as needed. Arms can rest at the sides, palms facing the ceiling.

Hold for 1 to 3 minutes (a).

Blanket backbend: Start from a seated position with the knees bent and feet on the mat. Place a rolled blanket behind the body across the mat. Position the blanket so that it is under the thoracic spine (midback, at the base of the shoulder blades) when you lie back on it.

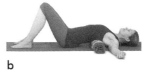

b

On the exhalation, gently lie back into the support of the blanket. Keep the knees bent and feet on the mat. Straighten the legs onto the floor, or bring the soles of the feet together and the knees out to the side in a butterfly shape.

The back of the head rests on the floor, or you can tuck a small rolled blanket under the curve of the back of the neck. Take your time to settle into the support of the pose and adjust as needed. Arms can rest out to the sides of the body on the floor at shoulder height with the palms facing the ceiling.

Hold for 1 to 3 minutes (b).

Side Bend

We spend a lot of our lives, and sometimes yoga practice, focused on the front or the back of the body and not quite as much on the sides. When you think of all of the ways the spine moves throughout the course of the day, lateral flexion is not often one of them.

The sides of the body are a powerful place for awareness. Especially because life comes with a lean for many people; they favor one side over the other, often the side of their dominant hand. Side bends are one of many opportunities you have to observe and work skillfully with the asymmetries of the body.

The great news is that once you start to pay attention to the lateral lines of the body, you may find that you use them more than you previously thought—especially if you play a sport like tennis, basketball, volleyball, or swimming. Awareness of the sides of the body also awakens new possibilities for breath and posture that can have an immediate and crucial impact on your stability in daily activities.

After differentiating your side bends, you may be surprised to find that the movement is smaller than you previously understood, especially when it is paired with a stable pelvis. Practitioners might develop a habit of accentuating their side bends with a forward bend or backbend or unnecessary hip movement in order to go deeper or farther into the movement. For that reason, it is important when differentiating side bends to play with variations that require you to focus on different aspects of the side bend so you can learn how to target certain areas without creating unnecessary movement in others. Happy side bending!

EXPLORATION

Side Bend

❶ Start by standing with the left arm long by the ear and the right hand on the right hip. Try to hold the pelvis in place and keep equal weight on the three points of each foot as you initiate the side bend evenly through the spine and arch to the right.

❷ Take a look at the left arm, side of the body, leg, and foot. Are they in line with each other or is the left arm in front of or behind the head? Can you sense whether you have brought a backbend, forward bend, or hip jut into the side bend?

❸ Focus on keeping space and length in both the elongated and shortened sides of the body. How does this initiation change your experience?

❹ Now stand against the wall in mountain pose. Heels can be slightly away from the wall as you make firm contact with the buttocks, shoulders, and back of the head against the wall. Arch into the side bend on both sides of the body as you maintain those back-of-body connections with the wall.

❺ Can you sense how the wall gives you valuable feedback on where your shoulders, spine, and torso are in relationship to your pelvis?

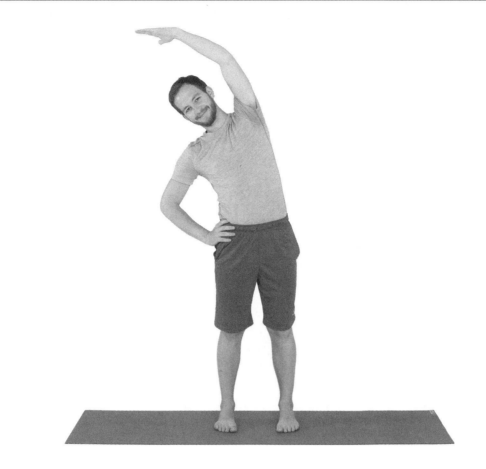

1. Start by standing with the feet hip-width apart. Bring the right hand to the right hip as you reach the left arm skyward. Arch the torso to the right. Ground yourself by applying pressure evenly into the triangle—big toe, pinky toe, center of the heel—on each foot.

2. As you hold the pose, maintain length in the side of the torso that is lengthening and in the side of the torso that is shortened. Use active support on the shortened side, resisting the temptation to collapse into the pose.

3. Hold for 30 to 90 seconds and repeat on the other side.

Basic Options

Bent elbows: Bend both elbows and place the hands at the base of the head, with the fingertips touching or the fingers interlaced to cup the head (a).

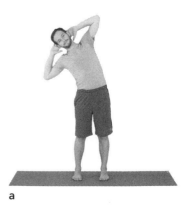

a

Upward reaching: Raise the arms out and up slightly above shoulder height with the palms facing forward. Draw a strap tautly between the hands. This variation can also be done with the arms by the ears, palms facing each other and the fingers interlaced above the head *(b)*.

Narrow base: Change the base of the pose by bringing the legs together, with the feet and legs touching *(c)*.

Bottom leg crossed: Cross the left leg in front of the right before arching to the right. Hold onto the left wrist with the right hand and gently lengthen the arm. Repeat on the other side, crossing the right leg in front of the left before arching to the left *(d)*.

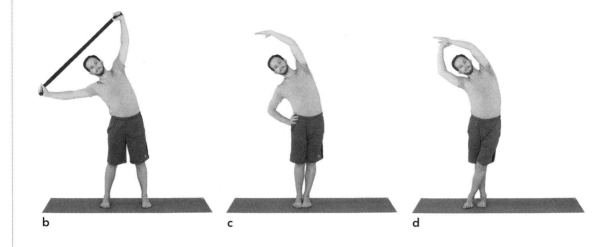

b   c   d

Mobility Option

At the wall: Turn the left side of the body toward the wall, 6 to 12 inches (15-30 cm) away from it. Reach the right arm up alongside the right ear, with the palm facing the wall. Arc toward the wall and press the right palm into the wall as you press the hand slightly upward without actually moving it. Hold 30 to 90 seconds. Repeat on the other side.

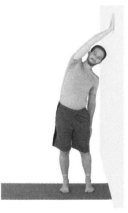

Strength Option

Weighted: Start in mountain pose, with the feet shoulders distance apart and holding 1- to 5-pound (.5-2.3 km) weights or sandbags in each hand. Use an inhalation to arch over to one side, maintaining pelvic stability as you move. On the exhalation, contract the lengthened side to help bring you back to center. Repeat on both sides 5 to 10 times.

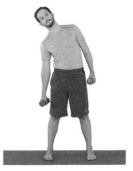

Reclined Side Bend

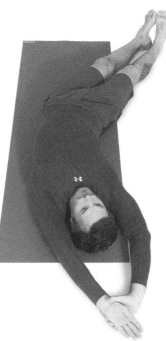

① Start in a fully reclined position with legs straight. Walk the legs over to the right (away from the midline of the body) a couple of inches (about 5 cm), keeping both buttocks in equal contact with the floor.

② Reach the arms up over the head and arch the upper body to the right, creating a crescent moon shape with the body, legs supported by the floor. Hold onto the left wrist with the right hand and give the arm a gentle lengthening pull.

③ Explore breathing into the rib cage on both sides of the torso as you hold the pose.

④ Hold for 1 to 2 minutes.

Basic Options

Crossed legs: Following the basic instructions, cross the left ankle on top of the right before arcing to the left. Switch sides, crossing the right ankle on top of the left before arcing right *(a)*.

Strap variation: Loop a strap over one of the feet (right foot if legs are uncrossed, left foot if legs are crossed) and bring it up outside of the right side of the body. Draw it taut with one or both hands above the head as you arch to the right *(b)*. Repeat on the other side.

Feet at the wall: Start in a fully reclined position, pressing both feet into the wall and keeping equal weight in both sides of the pelvis as it rests on the floor. Raise both arms above the head with the palms towards the ceiling, holding a strap and pulling it taught. Maintain the pull on the strap as you press both feet equally into the wall and arch the torso into a side bend. Repeat on the other side *(c)*.

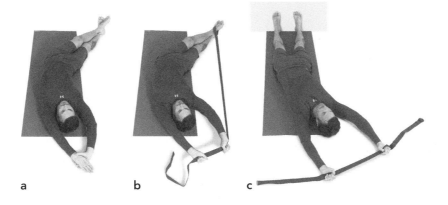

a   b   c

Twist

In daily life, twists help us see the world as we move through it. They allow us to see our surroundings while we are walking and driving and can be a source of tremendous power for our athletic endeavors—especially those that require us to throw or hit a ball. Yet, the ability to rotate is a skill that many of us lose as we age, which makes practicing rotation an important part of maintaining a healthy spine.

Done skillfully, twists offer valuable input to the soft-tissue structures that support the spine. As we free up some of the restrictions that we might encounter there, twists can help us find more grace and ease as we hold ourselves upright. They are a delightful way to break up a day of sitting if you are deskbound and can be used in a variety of ways to create balance in your yoga therapy practices.

The yoga world talks a lot about twists and detoxification. The image that is often used is that the organs of the body are like a sponge that we squeeze out and re-soak through the twisting action. This is not accurate. We don't really wring out or detoxify anything as a result of twisting. It is *movement itself* that is important. A body that moves in a variety of ways is a body that is more likely to flush itself. In this way, twists are just one aspect of a balanced movement practice that supports the body and all of its processes. We would suggest that the detox mantra of "rid the body of impurities" be replaced with the more body-positive mantra "I love and nourish my body through varied movement." Try it and see how it feels!

One of the foundations of skillful twisting is the ability to sense where the movement is happening in the spine. Generally speaking, we have the least amount of rotation available to us in the lumbar spine (low back), a little bit more in the thoracic spine (midback), and a whole lot in the cervical spine (neck).

Thoracic rotation tends to be difficult for people to find. One habit we often see is the tendency to either initiate the twist through the arms or to use the arms to pull the spine farther into the twist. It is also important to think about keeping the neck in line with the rest of the spine (all variations), the pelvis and feet grounded (standing and seated variations) and in contact with the floor. This helps focus the twist in the thoracic spine. The explorations will help you differentiate all of these aspects of the twist.

It is helpful to think of working in healthy ranges of motion and developing a combination of mobility, strength, and motor control on the way into the twist, during the hold, and on the way out. Use the arms to help you gently secure the position of the spine and work to uncover a healthy, unforced range of motion rather than using the arms to pull the spine into a twist. Happy twisting!

Twist

1 Stand with feet hip-width apart and the arms straight at your sides. Rotate to the right, allowing the pelvis to come forward as the left foot disconnects from the floor. Can you sense that while this might be a fun, free movement from side to side, not much spinal rotation occurs?

2 Return to center with both feet on the ground. Raise the arms out to the sides at shoulder height and the elbows bent at 90 degrees. Bring the spine into active neutral. Anchor the pelvis and the legs, keeping them still as you rotate through the spine to the right. Keep the head in line with the spine as you maintain equal weight on the three points in each foot throughout the twist. Only twist as far as you can while keeping the pelvis and legs active and still. Can you sense how this movement is more focused on the thoracic spine?

3 Perform the same twist, but from a seated position. Now glue the sits bones onto the floor and maintain equal weight on them as you twist. Can you sense how sitting and using the connection to the floor helps you to become more aware of maintaining a stable pelvis during focused thoracic rotation?

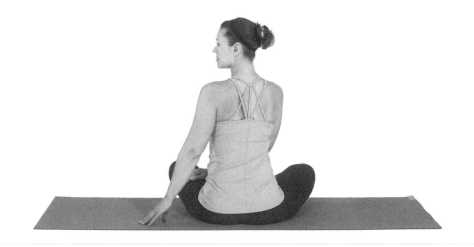

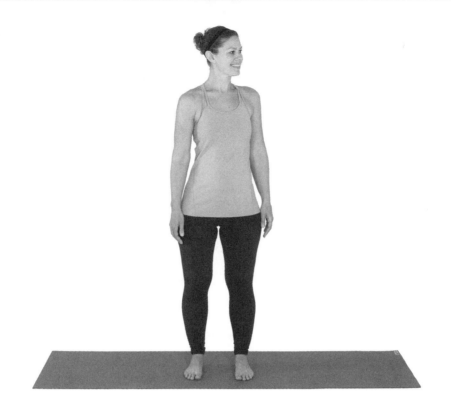

❶ Start by standing with the feet hip-width apart and the arms straight down at the sides, spine in active neutral.

❷ Keep the pelvis still and facing forward as you rotate the torso to the right on an exhalation while maintaining equal weight on both feet. Keep the head in line with the rest of the spine.

❸ Hold for 30 to 60 seconds and repeat on the other side.

Basic Option

Global twist: From standing with the feet hip-width apart and the arms by the sides, gently swing the torso, arms, and pelvis to the right, lifting the left foot as you rotate.

Come back through center and flow to the other side. Start slowly and build into a rhythmic movement as you become more comfortable in the flow.

Repeat 10 to 20 times, swinging from side to side.

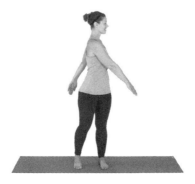

Strength Options

Flowing: From standing with the torso in active neutral, raise the arms to shoulder height with the elbows bent to 90 degrees and the palms facing forward.

Maintain active energy through the shoulders, arms, and hands, keeping them aligned as you rotate through the rib cage to the right, back to center, to the left, and back to center. As you move through the twist, keep the pelvis stable and maintain contact between the floor and all three points of each foot.

Repeat 10 to 20 times, rotating from side to side *(a)*.

Resistance band: You can also perform the flowing variation with the arms in front of the body just below shoulder height and a resistance band drawn taut between the hands *(b)*.

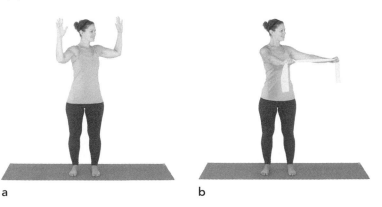

a   b

Balance Options

TIP: To help establish the balancing process before attempting it freestyle, perform variation 1 with the foot of the bent leg on a chair and variation 2 with the elevated leg straight and the foot pressed into the wall.

Single-leg variation 1: From standing, with the feet hip-width apart, bend the right knee so that the right thigh is in front of the pelvis. Ground the left foot by equally pressing all three points of the triangle—big toe, pinky toe, center of the heel—into the ground, and activate the standing leg. Raise the arms out to the sides at shoulder height.

Once you find your balance, rotate the torso toward the right leg.

Hold for 30 to 90 seconds, then slowly unwind to center and repeat on the other side *(a)*.

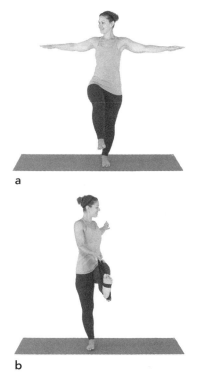

a

Single-leg variation 2: Position yourself the same as in variation 1, except now the bent knee is straight and the opposite hand is holding a strap taut around the arch of the foot as you rotate to towards the leg *(b)*. To add a strength challenge, try this version without the strap.

b

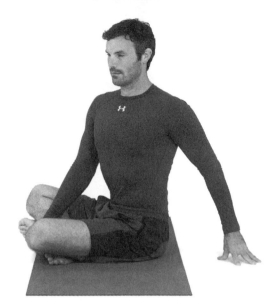

1. Start in a comfortable cross-legged seated position with the spine in active neutral and the arms at the sides of the body.

2. Keeping equal weight in the buttocks, exhale to initiate spinal rotation to the left, moving from the rib cage, allowing the shoulders, neck, head, and eyes to follow into the twist. Keep the head in line with the spine.

3. Place the right arm inside or outside of the right thigh and reach the left arm behind you, palm or fingertips on the floor. Resist the urge to use the arms to pull yourself farther into the pose.

4. Hold for 60 to 90 seconds and repeat on the other side.

Basic Options

Legs long: Extend both legs in front of you, pressing the heels forward and drawing the toes toward the face. Bend the elbows and bring the palms together in front of the chest. This variation can be done with the legs close together or wider apart *(a)*.

Asymmetrical: Start in a seated position with the right leg straight in front on the floor, the left knee bent, and the foot on the mat. Distribute weight equally on both sides of the pelvis. You can choose to place the left foot inside or outside of the right leg, closer or farther away from the pelvis. Rotate toward the leg with the bent knee, and hold for 30 to 60 seconds. Return to center and rotate away from the bent knee for another 30 to 60 seconds. Repeat on the other side *(b)*.

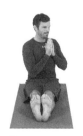

a

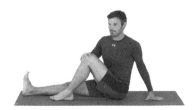

b

Mobility Option

At the wall: Sit on the floor with the legs crossed and right side of the body 4 to 6 inches (10-15 cm) away from the wall. Start with the spine in active neutral and equal weight in both buttocks.

Bend the elbows and position the arms in front of the body as you rotate toward the wall. Find your natural stopping point in the rotation without the help of the hands. Then place one or both palms on the wall to secure yourself in the twist.

Hold from 30 to 90 seconds and repeat on the other side.

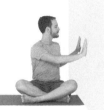

Strength Options

Hands free: From a cross-legged seated position, raise your arms out to the sides at shoulder height and the elbows bent at 90 degrees. The spine is in active neutral as you rotate through the rib cage, twisting only as far into the rotation as you can while keeping equal contact of both buttocks on the ground and without using your arms *(a)*.

Resistance twist: From a cross-legged seated position, secure the top of an exercise band under the right buttock in front of and across the body into the left hand. Raise the left arm to shoulder height or slightly lower with the palm facing forward and slightly angled toward the ceiling.

Keep the band taut and shoulder muscles active and steady as you rotate through the torso to the left *(b)*. This is a fluid exercise: Go slowly and control the rotation to the left and back to facing forward.

Repeat 10 to 20 times then switch the resistance band to under the left buttock and into the right hand. Repeat while rotating to the right.

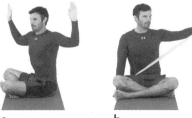

a   b

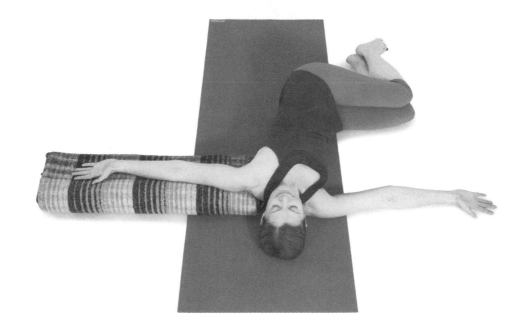

1. Start in a reclined position with the knees bent, feet on the floor, and the arms to the sides, resting on the floor at shoulder height with the palms up. Keep the inner legs and ankles glued together and let them move as a single unit with the pelvis to the right, resting on the floor or each other.

2. Maintain a connection between both shoulders and the ground. If the rotation is too intense, place a blanket or bolster between the legs and the floor to help reduce the amount of rotation.

3. The arms can settle on the floor at shoulder height, or the right hand can rest on the right thigh to help secure the twist. If the left shoulder pops off the ground, slide a folded blanket between it and the floor. Face the ceiling or rotate the neck to the left.

4. Hold 1 to 3 minutes and repeat on the other side.

Basic Options

Blanket supporting legs: Place a folded blanket between the bent knees to create a more relaxed sense of connection (a).

Legs long: Unbend the knees and bring the legs straight on the floor on top of each other, perpendicular to the torso (b).

Arm reach: Reach the left arm up by the ear instead of bringing it out at shoulder height (c).

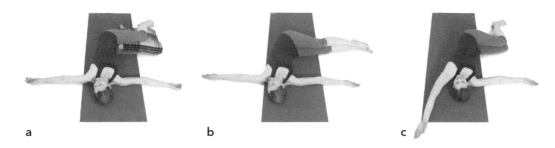

a

b

c

Strength Options

TIP: Where previous variations were a bit more passive, these variations actively engage the core. The first option is the easiest. Increase the challenge only if you are able to control the action on the way down and back to the starting position without using momentum.

Flowing variation 1: Start reclined with both knees bent and feet on the mat and arms out to the sides at shoulder height resting on the floor. Raise the feet off the mat and bring the shins in line with the knees as you stack thighbones in line with the pelvis. If needed, place a block between the bent knees and lightly press into it.

Exhale to rotate and bring the legs to the left side toward the floor without actually touching it. Inhale to unwind the trunk and bring the knees back to center.

Repeat 5 to 10 times from side to side *(a)*.

Flowing variation 2: Perform the same as variation 1, except the top leg lengthens to increase the challenge *(b)*.

Flowing variation 3: Perform the same as variation 2, except both legs lengthen to increase the challenge *(c)*.

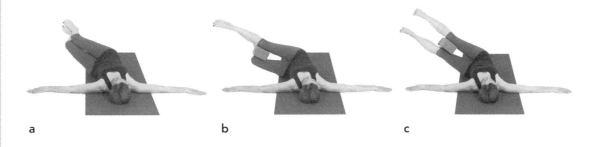

a   b   c

Recovery Option

Single leg with bolster: Start lying on the right side, the right leg straight on the floor in line with the pelvis, and foot relaxed on the floor. Bend the left knee and place it on a bolster or blanket stack.

Bring the arms out on the floor at shoulder height with the palms up. Exhale to initiate rotation from the center of the body to the left.

Hold for 1 to 3 minutes, then repeat on the other side.

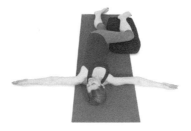

Now that you have identified, differentiated, and integrated the basic movements of the spine in a variety of orientations, it is time to gain new layers of experience as you explore the movements of the spine in more complex shapes. You will apply the skills that you have gained in this chapter to a whole new set of yoga pose categories in the next chapter. Enjoy applying your newly developed spinal awareness and seeing where it takes you in terms of an integrated experience of your personalized yoga therapy practices!

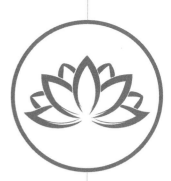

ten
Variations on Traditional Poses

In this chapter, you arrive at an interesting point on your journey of somatic inquiry. The process of **identification**, **differentiation**, and **integration** supported you in building a powerful foundation of movement skills, and the explorations that you have done thus far have opened up the possibility a whole new level of understanding. Here you will apply what you have learned in the previous chapters to basic yoga poses. And even though we use the word "basic" here, when you start to break them down, you will see there is really nothing basic about these shapes. They are designed to be fully integrated mind–body experiences, and your nervous system will definitely be challenged to solve a variety of new movement puzzles!

The poses in this chapter are divided into these categories: core, standing, balance, and hips. Although the categories are important as organizational structures, the ability to distinctly separate one category from another is more challenging at this point because they clearly overlap. For example, the poses in all of the categories require you to use your core in interesting ways. Any time you hold yourself upright, as in standing, there is an element of balance, so even the two-footed poses require interesting elements of balance. If you take a sweeping look at all of the poses in this book, you will see that some combination of hip mobility and stability is always present. In this way, your understanding of yoga poses can now expand into identifying, differentiating, and integrating the relationships between categories.

Take a moment to review what you have already learned about awareness, mindfulness, intention, breathing, and differentiated joint actions and how you applied those principles to the poses in the previous chapters. Now envision yourself expanding that knowledge base, continuing to explore all of those things within the context of new pose experiences. There are so many more possibilities ahead of you! Because we are unable to list every variation within the parameters of the written format, we are also asking you to use your experiences to expand on the potential of each pose. We encourage you to deviate from what we offer whenever you make a meaningful connection to something that has already come into your experiential sphere. Stay curious as you identify and differentiate what you have already learned, and look to integrate that knowledge with what you are exploring in this next section.

Core Poses

You might hear a lot of talk these days about the importance of the core. "Core strength" and "core stability" are just a few of the common terms that you have probably heard at some point in your yoga and fitness journey. The interesting thing is, that for all of the dialogue, there still doesn't seem to be universal agreement about what the core is. If you read and study for long enough, you will notice the definition of "core" tends to change based on the training method that you are exploring. Depending on what your goals are, you will have different experiences of the core, some of them more helpful or effective than others.

In fitness culture, the core is often the subject of certain aesthetic standards that are focused on the external show of some of the more superficial muscles of the core, known to many as six-pack abs. In reality, the core is a complex set of muscles that goes beyond the six-pack aesthetic: Functional core stability includes strength, endurance, flexibility, and motor control. Our approach moves away from attempting to train isolated core muscles in a single, held position or in one particular pelvic position. Instead we emphasize the various muscles that surround the core, including the abdominals, obliques, erector spinae, glutes, and pelvic floor and ask that you integrate core awareness into your favorite activities. We also like to emphasize the diaphragm as part of the core and remind you that while the diaphragm is one of the primary muscles of respiration, it is also a deep-core stabilizer. Using the breath differentiation exercises in tandem with the various movements of the spine highlighted in the previous chapters has already given you options for exploring your core in new and interesting ways.

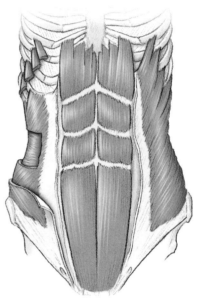

The muscles of the core.

Moving into this section, let's simplify the definition of the core as anything from below the end of the sternum and low borders of the rib cage to the base of the pelvis. This definition makes it easier to think about using yoga poses to make relevant connections from the upper and lower extremities into the core and explore different types of core activities in your yoga therapy practices. The next exploration revisits core activation as it relates to pelvic and spinal position along with basic pelvic floor and core activations. As always, variety is key.

Core Activation

1 Start in mountain pose. Place one hand on the abdomen and the other on the low back *(a)*.

2 Inhale to slowly roll the front of the pelvis toward the feet (anterior tilt), arching the low back *(b)*. Exhale to roll the front of the pelvis toward the face (posterior tilt), flattening the lumbar curve *(c)*. Notice how the tilt of the pelvis changes the sensation of the core muscles firing or not firing under your hands.

3 Roll the pelvis again, but reverse the breathing pattern, exhaling into the anterior tilt and inhaling into the posterior tilt. What, if anything, changes for you in terms of awareness?

4 Now move the pelvis and breathe at your natural rhythm, looking for equal muscular tension under both hands. When you find equal tension, you are approaching active neutral. Try to find a natural curve in the low back, where you are not overly arched or overly tucked.

5 From active neutral, try drawing up on the muscles of the pelvic floor, as if you are trying to stop the flow of urine. Hold the contraction for 30 seconds as you continue to breathe in the abdomen and rib cage.

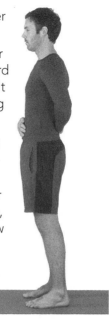

a

6 Now try drawing up on the muscles of the pelvic floor, as if you are trying to stop yourself from passing gas. Hold the contraction for 30 seconds as you continue to breathe in the abdomen and rib cage.

7 Draw up on both areas of the pelvic floor at the same time. Imagine zipping up into the low abdomen from the connection into the pelvic floor. Wrap that activity around to the low back. How does the awareness and core activation change as you make these new connections?

8 Now try working with both relaxing and contracting your pelvic floor, playing with increments of activation. Try drawing up on the pelvic floor 25, 50, 75, and 100 percent. Reverse and try to relax the pelvic floor down from 100 to 75, 50, and 25 percent. Play with how much activation is too much or too little as it relates to your ability to breathe, stabilize your core without being rigid, or holding on to the pelvic floor too tightly.

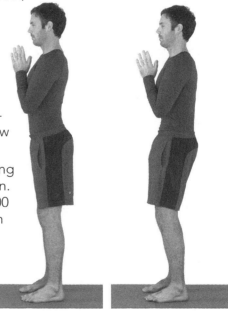

b   c

9 Now try steps 4 through 8 again, but with the spine in standing flexion (forward bend), extension (backbend), rotation (twist), and lateral flexion (side bend). How does your core awareness or activation change with the different positions of the spine?

10 Revisit the abdominal bracing and breathing technique from chapter 7 to get a sense of activating the inner abdominal corset and coordinating it with the breath. Continue to play with all of the concepts as you explore making meaningful core connections in the poses highlighted in this chapter.

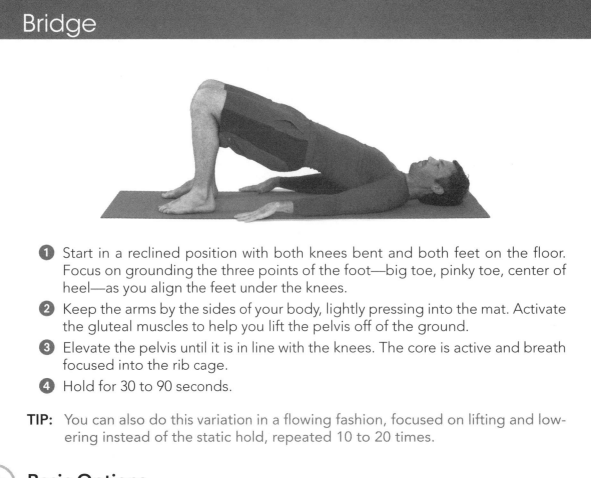

1. Start in a reclined position with both knees bent and both feet on the floor. Focus on grounding the three points of the foot—big toe, pinky toe, center of heel—as you align the feet under the knees.

2. Keep the arms by the sides of your body, lightly pressing into the mat. Activate the gluteal muscles to help you lift the pelvis off of the ground.

3. Elevate the pelvis until it is in line with the knees. The core is active and breath focused into the rib cage.

4. Hold for 30 to 90 seconds.

TIP: You can also do this variation in a flowing fashion, focused on lifting and lowering instead of the static hold, repeated 10 to 20 times.

Basic Options

TIP: For a mobility option, revisit the articulating bridge option from the spine series in chapter 8.

Block or ball between thighs: Place a small exercise ball or yoga block between the thighs. Give it a light squeeze and stay connected to all three parts of both feet as you lift, hold, and lower out of the pose (a).

Strap around thighs: Firmly loop a strap around the outside of the thighs. Lightly press into the feedback of the strap and stay connected to all three parts of both feet as you lift, hold, and lower out of the pose (b).

Balls and heels of feet: Come into the basic bridge shape and lift the heels off the ground for the duration of the hold (c). Lower the heels back to the ground before coming out of the shape. Repeat with the balls of the feet slightly lifted and the heels on the ground (d).

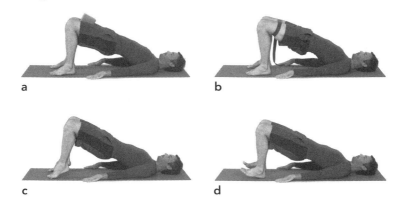

a

b

c

d

Strength Options

Single-leg variation: Lift the left leg in line with the right thigh. With an inhalation, firmly press the right foot into the floor and lift the pelvis off the ground. With an exhalation, slowly lower the pelvis back to the ground. Repeat 5 to 10 times and then perform on the other side. This variation can also be done as a static hold for 30 to 60 seconds on each side *(a)*.

Marching bridge: Follow the instructions for a basic bridge, but instead of holding the pose static at the top, lift one foot at time 1 inch (2.5 cm) off of the ground and put it back down slowly, alternating feet. Repeat 5 to 10 times alternating on each side *(b)*.

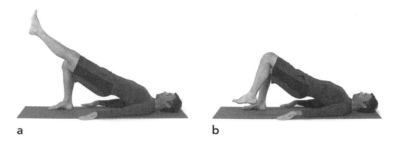

a   b

Balance Option

On a ball: Start in a reclined position with the legs straight and the heels and calves resting on a large exercise ball. Exhale to slowly articulate the pelvis and midspine off of the ground and into a bridge shape. Hold anywhere for 10 to 30 seconds at the top and then slowly articulate the midspine then lower spine back to the mat. Repeat 5 to 10 times.

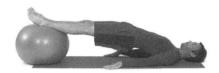

Recovery Option

Supported bridge: Place a yoga block on the low (long and wide) or medium (long and narrow) setting under the low back. Knees may remain bent and feet on the mat, or you can try sliding one or both legs straight with the heels resting on the floor. Arms can stay by the sides of the body or reach up by the ears. Hold for 1 to 3 minutes.

TIP: If the block placement in this variation causes a pinching sensation in the low back or is uncomfortable, move it up or down an inch or two (2.5-5 cm) to find a sweet spot of support. You can also try a lower setting, or replace the block with a firm, rectangular bolster or Z-folded blanket.

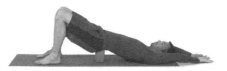

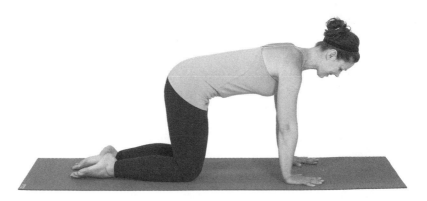

1. Start on all fours with the hands under the shoulders and knees under the hips. Bring the thighbones in line with the knees, keeping space between them. The tops of the feet are on the mat, palms are on the ground, arms are straight, and fingertips are pointing forward.

2. The spine is in active neutral, supported by a slight abdominal engagement.

3. Hold for 30 to 60 seconds.

Basic Options

Wrist option: To reduce wrist flexion, roll up the top of your mat or a small towel to place under the heels of the hands (a).

Foot option: Place the balls of the feet instead of the tops of the feet on the mat. Use this version if you get foot cramps in the basic position (b).

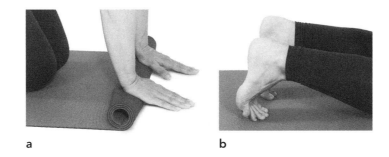

a   b

Mobility Options

Table twist: Exhale to rotate through the torso to the right, reaching the right arm skyward. Exhale to pass through the center and rotate left as you reach the right arm across the front of the body. Repeat 5 to 10 times in a flowing fashion (a and b). On the last repetition, with the left arm across the front of the body, bring the left shoulder and side of the face to rest on the floor. Walk the right arm toward the front of the mat with the palm pressed firm into the floor. Hold for 30 to 90 seconds and repeat on the other side (c).

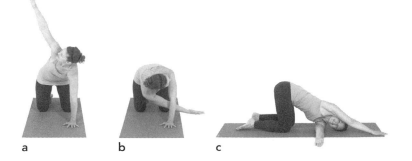

a   b   c

Table side-bend variation 1: Exhale to bring the right shoulder and the right hip toward each other. Inhale to come back to center, and exhale to the other side. Repeat 5 to 10 times.

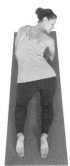

Table side-bend variation 2: Keep the pelvis fixed and level as you walk the hands and torso to the right a few inches (about 5 cm) and arch into a side bend. Hold for 30 to 60 seconds. Come back to the starting position and walk the hands and torso over to the left side, holding the pose on the left for an equal amount of time.

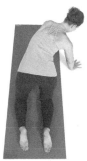

Hip drop: Bring the knees together in table. Exhale and shift the pelvis toward the floor on the right. Inhale to bring the pelvis back to center. Repeat on the left and continue, creating a fluid motion side to side that matches your breath. Repeat 10 to 20 times.

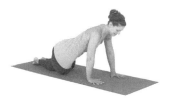

Strength Options

Fire hydrant: Lift the right hip and knee out to the right side, keeping the pelvis as parallel to the floor as possible, maintaining active neutral in the spine *(a)*. Hold for 30 to 60 seconds, and then repeat on the other side.

Flying table: Turn the toes under and press into the balls of the feet to lift the knees an inch or two (2.5-5 cm) off the floor. Press the hands into the mat and spread the shoulder blades apart *(b)*. Pull the hands lightly back toward the feet without actually moving them. Hold for 30 to 60 seconds.

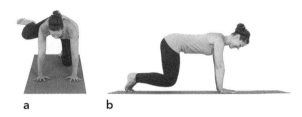

a   b

Balance Options

Balancing table variation 1: From table, lift the left arm and right leg off of the ground, keeping them in line with the shoulder and pelvis *(a)*. Maintain active neutral in the spine. Hold for 30 to 60 seconds, and then repeat on the other side.

Balancing table variation 2: From variation 1, take the left arm out to the left and the right leg out to the right *(b)*. Hold for 30 to 60 seconds, and then repeat on the other side.

Balancing table variation 3: From variation 1 or variation 2, try drawing small circles with the lifted arm and leg. Repeat 5 to 10 times and then circle in the other direction.

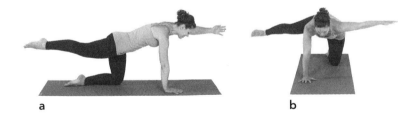

a   b

Downward-Facing Dog

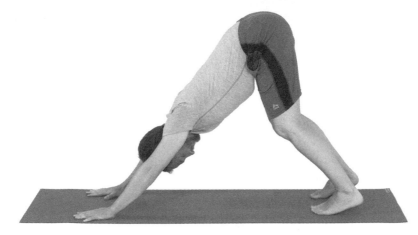

❶ From hands and knees, relax the hands and let the fingertips open to the floor in a natural cupped position. Lightly press the hands into the floor as you elevate the pelvis toward the ceiling, coming into an upside down V-shape.

❷ Keep the knees bent, find a natural lumbar curve, and play with walking the feet out and pressing the heels toward the ground. When you have found a stable position, straighten the knees only if you can keep the spine and pelvis in an active-neutral position.

❸ Spread the shoulder blades and draw them down toward the top of the pelvis, keeping equal weight on both hands.

❹ Hold for 30 to 90 seconds.

Basic Options

Forearm variation 1: Bend the elbows and place the forearms and palms onto the floor (a).

Forearm variation 2: Bend the elbows and place the sides of the forearms and pinkie-finger edge of the hands onto the mat. Press the palms into the sides of a block placed in the low setting (flat and horizontal) between the hands (b).

Feet supported by blanket: Place a small rolled blanket under the heels of both feet (c).

Feet together: Bring the feet and legs together so that the legs touch. You could also lightly squeeze a block or small exercise ball between the upper thighs (d).

Feet apart: Walk the feet and legs shoulder-width apart or wider. If wider than shoulder-width, turn to the long edge of the mat so that you have the space to bring the feet and legs 2 to 3 feet (61-91 cm) apart (e).

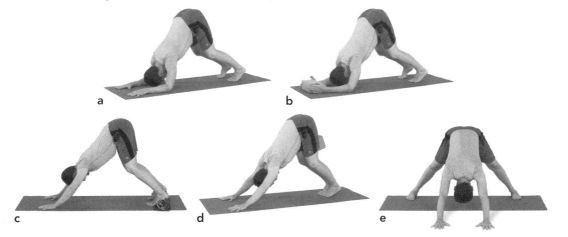

a

b

c

d

e

Mobility Options

Walking-dog variation 1: From the basic position, bend the knees and walk the feet toward the hands, stopping just before you get to a bent-knee forward fold. Slowly walk the feet and spine back into downward-facing dog. Repeat 5 to 10 times.

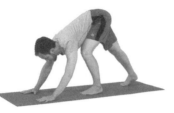

Walking-dog variation 2: Bend the knees and walk the hands toward the feet, stopping just before you get to a bent-knee forward fold. Slowly walk the hands and spine back into downward-facing dog. Repeat 5 to 10 times.

Balance Options

Single-leg variation 1: From the basic position, lift the left leg in line with the pelvis (a).

Single-leg variation 2: From variation 1, bend the left knee. Keep the upper body stable as you rotate through the torso to the left, opening the left hip out to the side (b).

Asymmetrical variation 1: Elevate both feet on blocks set on the long, flat setting (c).

Asymmetrical variation 2: Elevate both hands on blocks set on the long, flat setting (d).

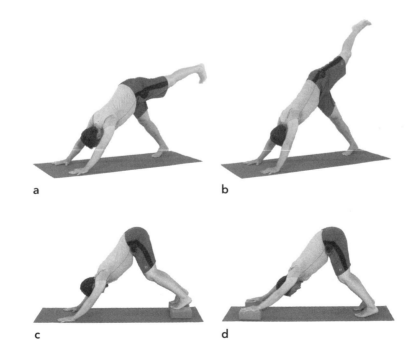

a

b

c

d

Boat

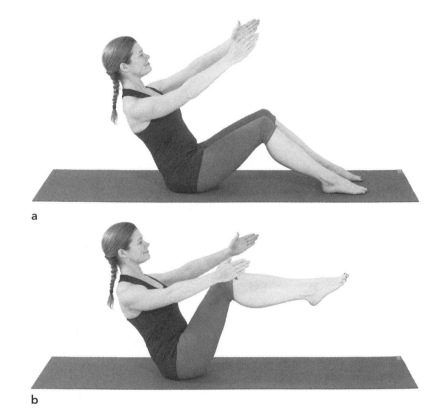

a

b

1. Start in a seated position with the knees bent, feet on the floor, and the spine upright in active neutral.

2. Reach the arms forward at shoulder height, and engage a light abdominal brace as you hinge back from the hips to a 45-degree angle with the torso (a).

3. Keep the feet on the ground or, for more challenge, lift the soles of the feet off the ground and bring the lower legs in line with the knees (b). Maintain equal weight in both buttocks. Keep the knees bent or, to increase the challenge, start to straighten the legs. Only straighten the legs if you can maintain abdominal stability and keep the spine in active neutral.

4. Hold for 30 to 60 seconds.

Basic Options

Hands or strap on back of the thighs: Place both hands on the backs of the thighs to help find balance and stability (a). If needed, extend the reach of the arms by looping a strap behind the thighs and drawing it taut with the hands.

At the wall: Place the bottom of both feet against the wall about hip-width apart. This variation can be done with the knees bent or straight (b).

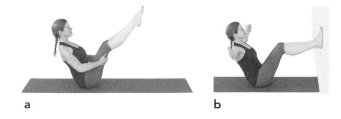

a

b

Arms by the sides: Arms comes slightly behind the torso with the elbows bent and palms on the floor *(c)*.

Elbows bent: Fingers interlace behind the head and the elbows point out from the sides of the body *(d)*. This variation can also be done with the backs of the hands touching the forehead if behind the head is too much for the neck or shoulders.

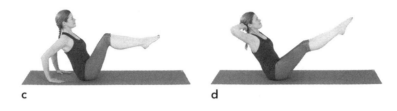

c   d

Mobility Alternative

Articulating boat: Start in a reclined position with the knees bent and feet on the mat. Exhale, bring the chin toward the chest, reach the arms forward, and slowly articulate the spine through roundness as you come to upright *(a and b)*. The arms are raised by the ears and the spine comes through active neutral and then into a small thoracic-focused backbend *(c)*. Bring the arms forward, and exhale to reverse the articulation, lowering the pelvis and then spine to the floor. Repeat 5 to 10 times.

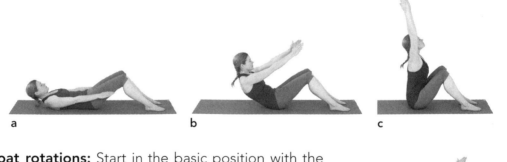

a   b   c

Boat rotations: Start in the basic position with the feet grounded or lifted. Keep equal weight on both buttocks as you exhale to rotate to the right, inhale back to center, exhale to rotate left, and inhale back to center. Repeat 10 to 20 times *(d)*.

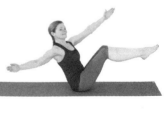

d

Strength Alternative

Low boat: Start in a reclined position with the legs together and pointing sky-ward. Exhale, bring the chin toward the chest, reach the arms forward, and slowly articulate the upper spine into roundness, slightly flattening the low back into the ground and creating a C-shape with the upper half of the body. Keep the legs straight and experiment with lowering them toward the floor. The closer the legs get to the floor, the more difficult it will be to maintain abdominal stability. Hold for 30 to 60 seconds.

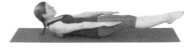

Standing Poses

At some time in your life you have probably heard that good posture is important. Perhaps you had a parent who encouraged you to stand up straight to show respect or a teacher who told you to stop slouching as a way to affirmatively present yourself to the world. Yet the ability to skillfully hold the spine upright requires a level of awareness and finesse that is on the decline. The technological age has proven challenging for the average human's postural habits.

Posture is more relevant to our life experience than we could have imagined as kids. It would have been nice if our parents and teachers had explained that it's important because it is so much more than just standing up straight. Healthy posture has been proven to positively affect the ability to breathe. As the ability to breathe improves, all of the systems of the body benefit in some way, especially the digestive and circulatory systems. Wear and tear on the musculoskeletal system can be lessened through the practice of healthy posture, which increases muscular efficiency while decreasing unnecessary joint deterioration. It is important to note that healthy upright posture does not mean that you have to make your body stiff or rigid, as in military style. Healthy posture is adaptable to the situation you are in and demonstrates an ability to use the spine along with the rest of the body in a way that is optimal for the activity that you are trying to accomplish.

Healthy posture also lessens positional stress on the nervous system, which can lead to a host of unexpected benefits as you age, including improved range of motion, decreased pain, increased lung capacity, and a more outwardly youthful appearance. It also affects how others view you; other people's perception of your posture can influence your success or failure when you attempt certain interactive feats, such as finding a job or making an important speech.

Outside of adept breathing, the ability to skillfully hold your spine upright is one of the most important functional outgrowths of a personalized yoga therapy practice. This is one of the reasons we have spent so much time exploring mountain pose in this book. Mountain pose is the solid foundation from which you can successfully build all of your other standing poses. The next section offers new and interesting ways for you to continue to cultivate the ability to skillfully hold your spine upright in yoga practice and daily activities.

Postural Connections

① Review the mountain pose inquiry in chapter 5. This next exploration applies some of the foundational postural concepts that you explored in that section of warrior 1.

② Stand in your favorite variation of warrior 1. Pay special attention to the relationship between your feet, pelvis, spine, shoulders, and head. Where is your center of gravity in this position? How much effort or relaxation are you using to hold yourself upright?

③ Notice where the effort is necessary and helpful and where it drains your energy. What is the difference between rigid and active? What is the difference between strategically relaxed and lazy or sloppy?

④ Now make your intention efficiency or economy of effort without being lazy. How does that change the effort or relaxation aspects of your posture? How does it feel if you lengthen yourself toward the ceiling, as if being pulled by a string on top of your head?

⑤ Explore the movement of your pelvis in this posture. Play with slowly articulating the pelvis into a small posterior tilt (tucked) and anterior tilt (untucked) position. When you find active neutral in the spine, pay attention to how that affects the experience of your posture.

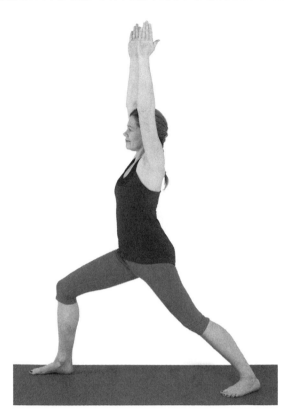

⑥ Explore your spine in the posture. Try out flexion (forward bend), extension (backbend), rotation (twist), and lateral flexion (side bend). How does your postural awareness change with the position of the spine?

⑦ Explore your feet in this posture. Pay special attention to what happens to your posture when you connect all three points the foot—big toe, small toe, center of heel—into the floor.

⑧ Now activate the legs by pulling the mat together with the feet without actually doing so. Activate the legs by attempting to pull the feet away from each other without actually moving them, as if you were going to rip your mat apart. How do these intentions for muscular engagement change your experience?

⑨ Try layering in breath and core activations from the explorations in the previous section. How do they change your experience of holding yourself upright? Continue to explore these layers of awareness as you move on to the poses highlighted in this section.

Chair

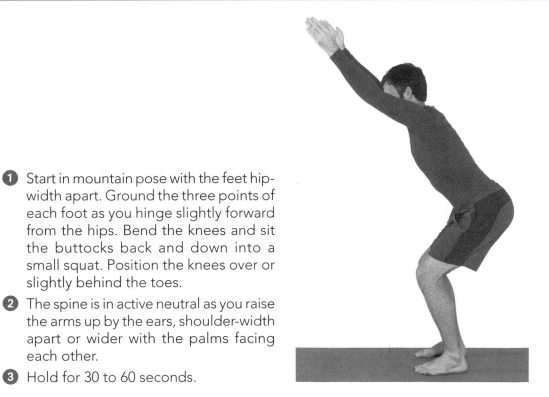

1. Start in mountain pose with the feet hip-width apart. Ground the three points of each foot as you hinge slightly forward from the hips. Bend the knees and sit the buttocks back and down into a small squat. Position the knees over or slightly behind the toes.

2. The spine is in active neutral as you raise the arms up by the ears, shoulder-width apart or wider with the palms facing each other.

3. Hold for 30 to 60 seconds.

Basic Options

Narrow base: Bring the feet and legs together so they touch. Work on staying connected to all three points of the foot in the narrower base of support *(a)*.

Wide base: Position the legs 2 to 3 feet (61-91 cm) apart with the toes slightly turned out to the sides *(b)*.

Arms by the side of the body: Position the arms along the sides of the body with the palms facing the legs. Reach actively through the arms *(c)*.

Palms together: Press the palms lightly together in front of the chest *(d)*.

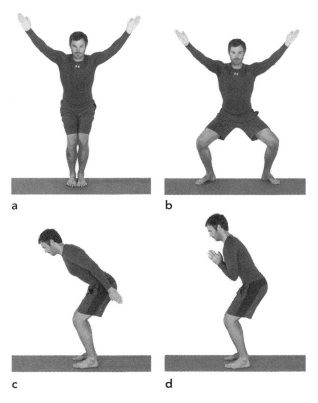

a

b

c

d

Mobility Options

Rotation: Start in the basic position arms out to the side at shoulder height. Place the ends of a strap or exercise band in each hand, pulling it taut across the chest. Exhale to rotate through the midspine to the left, keeping the arms straight and strap taut as you go. Keep equal weight on the three points of each foot as you move. Inhale to return to center. Repeat 5 to 10 times, moving side to side. You can also do this variation without the strap *(a)*.

Cat–cow chair: Start in the basic position with the arms out to the side at shoulder height and hands in gentle fists. Exhale and roll the fists downward, initiating the movement from the shoulders, allowing the upper spine to follow into a small upper abdominal curl *(b)*. Inhale and roll the fists away from the floor, initiating the movement from the shoulders, articulating the spine back to neutral and then into a small thoracic-focused backbend *(c)*. Repeat 5 to 10 times.

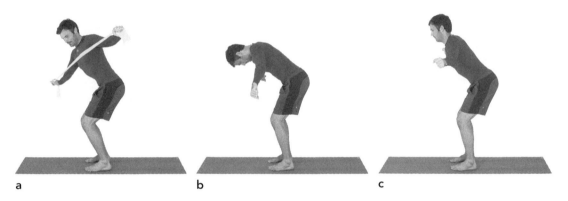

a   b   c

Strength Options

Strap: Start in the basic position, holding a strap in both hands above the head. Pull the strap as the shoulders slightly depress. Hold for 30 to 60 seconds *(a)*.

At the wall: Stand with the back of the body against the wall. Walk the feet out, bending the knees to approximately 90 degrees. The shins and feet are aligned under the knees. Keep the spine upright in active neutral as you connect to the wall. Bring the arms out to the sides at shoulder height with the elbows bent at 90 degrees against the wall and the palms facing forward. Hold for 30 to 60 seconds *(b)*.

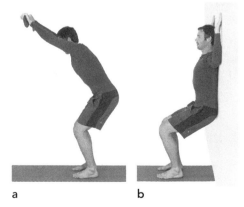

a   b

Balance Options

Balancing chair variation 1: Start by standing with the left foot on a wide, long, flat yoga block with the arms out to the sides at shoulder height. Line up the toes of both feet next to each other and the feet hip-width apart. Bend the left knee, leveling the pelvis. To more skillfully work with the asymmetrical base that you have created, lessen the degree that you bend the knees and sink the hips back. Hold for 30 to 60 seconds, and then repeat on the other side (a).

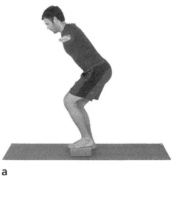

a

Balancing chair variation 2: Start in the basic chair position with arms out to the sides at shoulder height. Lift one foot a few inches (about 5 cm) off of the floor while maintaining active neutral in the spine. Hold for 30 to 60 seconds, and then repeat on the other side (b).

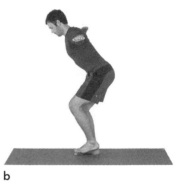

b

Balancing chair variation 3: Stand with the heels lifted off the ground, balancing on the balls of the feet. Bring the hands together in front of the chest. Bend the knees and squat only as far as you can maintain the connection through the entire ball of the foot and then return to standing without assistance. Return to standing either on the balls of the feet or with the heels down to assist in the motion. Hold for 30 to 60 seconds (c).

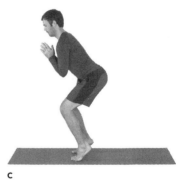

c

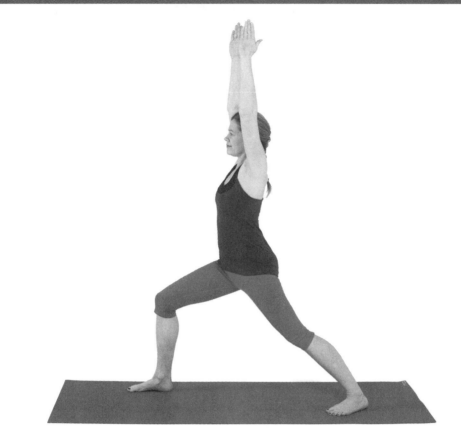

1. Start by standing with the feet hip-width apart. Keep the right leg forward as you step the left leg back and place the left foot on the ground behind you. Space the legs as if standing on railroad tracks about 1 to 2 feet (30-61 cm) apart.

2. Bend the right knee, connecting into all three points of both feet, as you activate the back leg. The back foot is on the ground behind the torso with the foot and pelvis turned slightly out toward the edge of the mat.

3. The spine stays in active neutral as you reach the arms up near the ears, with the palms facing each other.

4. Hold for 30 to 90 seconds and repeat on the other side.

Basic Options

Wide vs. narrow base: Play with decreasing the distance between the front and back leg (a).

Heel lifted vs. grounded: From the basic position, shift the pelvis slightly forward as you pivot on the ball of the back foot and disconnect the back heel from the ground. Keep the ball of the back foot equally connected to the ground from the big toe to the pinky toe as you hold the pose (b).

Arm position variation 1: Start in the basic position, with hands on the hips (c).

Arm position variation 2: Start in the basic position and raise the left arm above the head, while the right arm is down along the side of body (d).

Back foot at the wall: Press the heel of the back foot into the wall (e).

Front knee at the wall: Place a yoga block between your front knee and the wall. Use the feedback of the block and light pressure from the knee to pin the block to the wall (f).

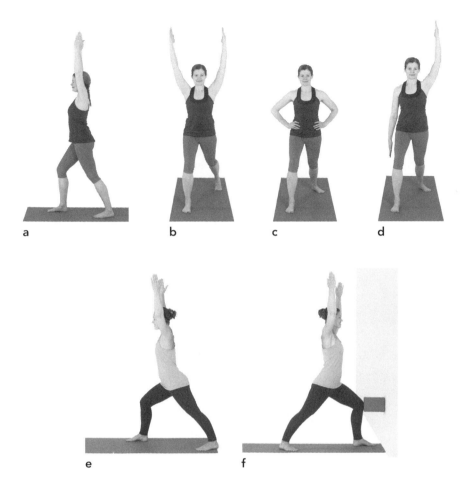

a   b   c   d

e   f

Mobility Options

Spinal flexion: Start in the basic position with the arms straight behind the body, palms facing skyward, and holding a strap taut. Round the spine toward the thigh, allowing the arms to float up toward the head as you fold forward (a).

Cat–cow: Start in the basic position with the arms out to the sides at shoulder height and the hands in gentle fists facing skyward. Exhale and roll the fists downward, initiating the movement from the shoulders and allowing the upper and midspine to follow into a small C-curve (b). Inhale, rolling the fists away from the floor, initiating the movement from the shoulders as you articulate the spine back to neutral and then into a small thoracic-focused backbend (c). Repeat 5 to 10 times.

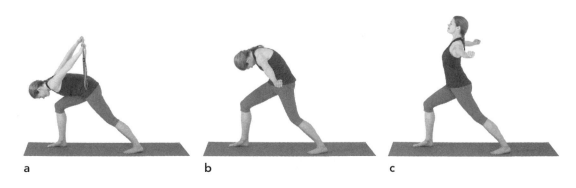

a   b   c

Spinal rotation: Start in the basic position with the arms out to the sides and the elbows bent at a 90-degree angle. Maintain a level pelvis, connect all three points of both feet into the floor as you rotate to the right, rotate to the left, and return to center. Repeat 5 to 10 times. You can also do this variation with the arms out to the sides at or just below shoulder height, pulling a yoga strap or exercise band taut *(d)*.

Lateral flexion: Start in the basic position with the arms down at the sides of the body. Reach the right arm up over the head. Slide the left arm and hand down the side of the body toward the floor as you arch the spine to the left. Come back to center, switch which arm is up and arch the spine to the right, this time with the left leg forward. This variation could also be done with both arms up, hands together, or apart *(e)*.

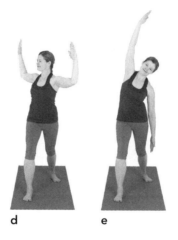

d   e

Strength Options

Hip flexion with spine in active neutral: From the basic position, hinge forward from the hips to bring the torso to roughly 45 degrees, hovering over the right thigh *(a)*. This variation can also be done with the arms out to the sides at shoulder height or reaching long by the ears.

Exercise band variation 1: Position an exercise band under the ball of the front foot, holding the ends taut in each hand with the arms down toward the floor. Bend both elbows, keeping the upper arms in line with the torso and wrists in line with the forearms as you pull the band towards the torso. Exhale to straighten the elbows back into the starting position. Repeat 10 to 15 times *(b)*.

Exercise band variation 2: Position an exercise band under the ball of the front foot, holding the ends taut in each hand with the arms down toward the front foot. Exhale to bend both elbows, pulling on the band as the elbows move out to the sides of the body into a square shape. Inhale to straighten the elbows and bring the arms back into the starting position. Repeat 10 to 15 times *(c)*.

Exercise band variation 3: Position an exercise band under the ball of the front foot, holding the ends in each hand, with the arms long toward the front knee. Keep the arms straight and the wrists in line with the forearms as you pull the band and sweep the arms behind the body. Inhale to bring the arms back to the starting position. Repeat 10 to 15 times *(d)*.

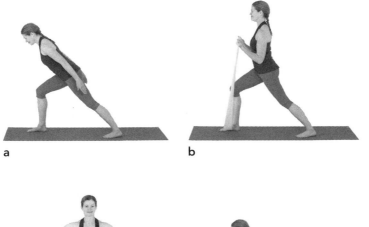

a

b

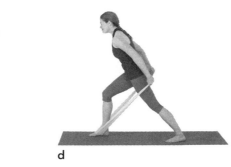

c

d

Balance Option

Back foot on block: Place the back foot on a block on the low setting (long and flat) on the floor.

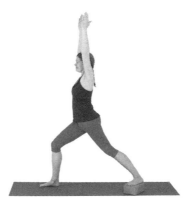

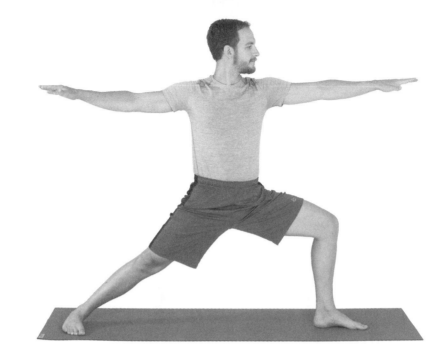

1. Start in mountain. Keep the left foot forward as you open the right hip and pelvis to the right and step the right foot to the back of the mat. Heels of the front and back feet can either line up or have up to 6 inches (15 cm) of space between them (as if standing on railroad tracks instead of a balance beam). Arms come out to a T-shape at shoulder height with palms down.

2. Bend the front knee and connect all three points of the front foot into the ground. Activate the back leg and ground all three points of the back foot. Play with the back hip and foot position: turned slightly in, parallel, and slightly out. The spine can stay in active neutral for the duration of the hold.

3. Hold for 30 to 90 seconds, and repeat on the other side.

Basic Options

Wide vs. narrow base: Play with decreasing the distance between the front and back leg (a).

Arms variation 1: Start in the basic position, with hands on the hips (b).

Arms variation 2: Start in the basic position with the back arm raised above the head and the front arm straight out in front at shoulder height (c).

Front knee at the wall: Place a yoga block horizontally between your front knee and the wall. Use the feedback of the block and light pressure from the knee to pin the block to the wall (d).

Back of the body at the wall: Using the basic position for warrior 2, bring the back of the body to the wall, letting the wall to help create more postural awareness (e).

Front arm at the wall: Hold a block in the front hand on the short end. Press the other end of the block into the wall (f).

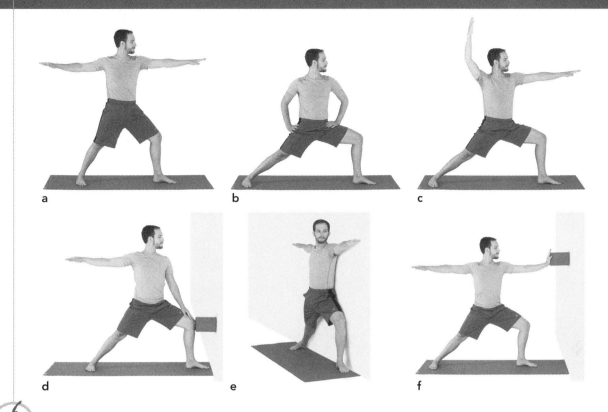

a   b   c

d   e   f

Mobility Options

Cat–cow: Start in the basic position with the arms out to the side at shoulder height with the palms facing skyward. Exhale to roll the palms toward the ground, initiating the movement from the shoulders and allowing the spine to actively round (a). Inhale, then roll the palms away from the floor, initiating the movement from the shoulders as you articulate the spine back to neutral and then into a small backbend (b). Repeat 5 to 10 times.

Rotation: Start in the basic position with the arms wide and slightly in front of body at shoulder height or just below, drawing a yoga strap or exercise band taut. Maintain a level pelvis and ground all three points of each foot as you rotate to the right and left. Repeat 10 to 15 times. You can also do this variation without the exercise band, elbows bent at 90 degrees, or straight and active out to the sides at shoulder height (c).

Lateral flexion: Start in the basic position with the arms along the sides of the body. Reach the front arm up and active. Slide the back arm hand down the back leg, arching the spine back as you go. Repeat with the opposite leg forward (d).

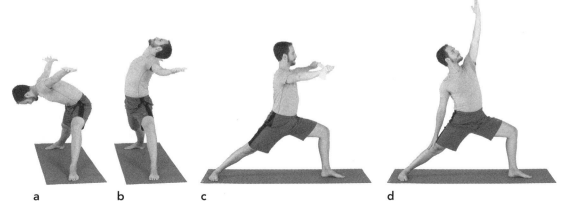

a   b   c   d

Strength Option

Exercise band: Start in the basic position with the end of the band under the back foot. Hold onto the other end with the front hand, keeping the forearm across the torso and the shoulder internally rotated *(a)*. Keeping the elbow bent, open the arm out to the side into external rotation, and then straighten and reach it forward and up (shoulder height or just below) *(b)*. The back arm is out to the side at shoulder height for the duration of the hold. Reverse the movements back to center, repeat 5 to 10 times, and then on the other side.

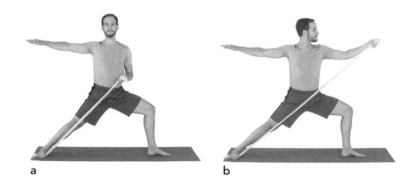

a   b

Balance Option

Front foot on block: Place the front foot on a block set on its low setting (long and flat) on the floor underneath the foot.

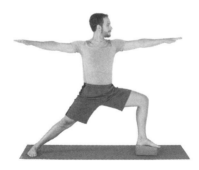

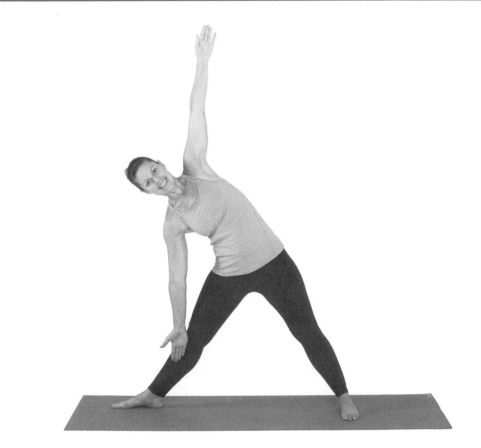

1. Start in warrior 2 with the right leg forward and the arms out to the sides at shoulder height. Straighten the front leg. Reach the front arm and torso over the front leg. Arch from the spine to bring the torso toward the thigh, maintaining length on both sides of the torso.

2. Lightly touch the right hand to the thigh or shin of the front leg. Keep the core active and resist the urge to sink into the support of the hand.

3. Stack the left arm over the shoulder and reach skyward. Keep the neck in line with the spine and the head facing forward.

4. Hold for 30 to 60 seconds.

Basic Options

Wide vs. narrow stance: Play with decreasing or increasing the distance between the front and back leg. Note that the model is in active neutral spinal position to demonstrate the change in stance (a and b).

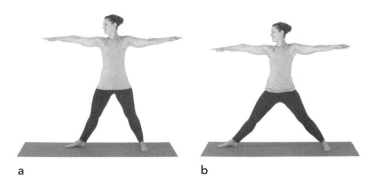

a   b

Front knee bends: Play with the degree of bend in the knee, from very small to 90 degrees *(c)*. This variation can be practice with the front forearm on the thigh (as pictured) or explored in tandem with any of the other arm variations.

Arm variation 1: Bend the top arm and place the hand at the hip *(d)*.

Chair or block: Place the lower arm or hand on the seat of a chair or onto a block placed outside or inside of the front leg. Play with the distance between the chair or block and your foot *(e)*.

Wall: Using the basic variation, make contact between the back of the body and the wall to help create more postural awareness *(f)*.

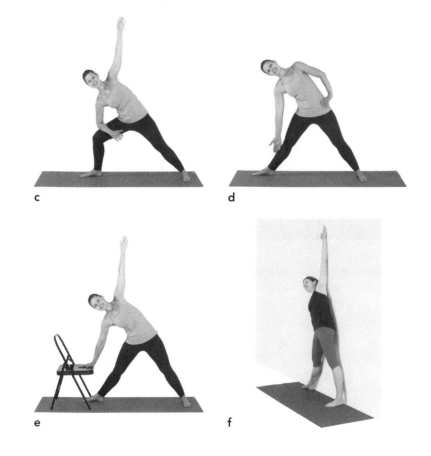

c

d

e

f

Mobility Option

Flowing: Start in the bent knee variation. Exhale to sweep the upper arm back towards the feet *(a)*, and then rotate the torso down toward the ground as you reach the arm forward *(b)*. Inhale and sweep up and back toward the starting position.

Keep equal weight on the three points of each foot as you explore the movement. Repeat 5 to 10 times and then flow the arm and torso in the opposite direction before trying it on the other side.

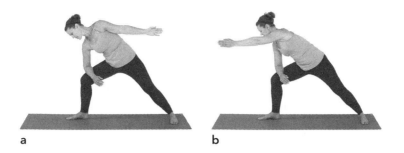

a   b

Strength Options

Strap pull: Start in the basic position with the arms out to the sides at shoulder height, holding a strap taut between them. As you enter the pose, instead of placing the right hand on the leg or a block, perform the pose without the support of the right arm and hand (a).

Hands free: Start in the basic position with the arms raised above the head and slightly away from the ears (b). As you enter into the pose, keep the arms in this position and do the pose without the support of the lower arm or hand.

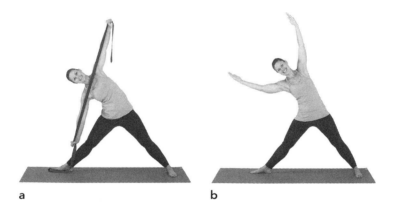

a   b

Balance Alternatives

Neck position: In any of the variations, keep the neck in line with the spine as you turn the head to look down at the ground (a) or up at the sky (b). Neck position options are demonstrated in the asymmetrical variation.

Asymmetrical variation: Place the right foot on a block on the horizontal (flat) setting. Use another block on the high setting under the right hand (a and b).

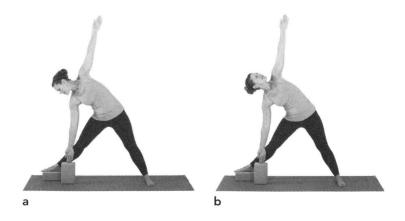

a   b

Balance Poses

At this point in your explorations, you are no stranger to the physical intention of balance in practice. You have been cultivating your ability to balance in a variety of orientations and spinal positions and have challenged your nervous system with asymmetrical and cross-body movement patterns designed to increase your ability to sense where your body is in space. The physical benefits of exploring balance in your yoga therapy practices have probably already carried over into other life pursuits. Balance is an important element in any sport because you will not perform your sport very well if you fall down all the time! Any martial artist will tell you that balance and awareness are the keys to generating power.

Balance is also important in your everyday activities. Whenever you lose your balance, the quicker you can regain it, the safer your movement will be. Every year 2.8 million older Americans are treated in emergency rooms for fall-related injuries (CDC 2016). It is unclear exactly how many of those falls lead to death, but the loss of quality of life or potential for diminished capacity of movement after recovery is significant for many people. That means that proactively improving your balance and increasing your proprioception may actually improve your overall quality of life along with prolonging life itself. To successfully practice balance, you also have to explore falling. We suggest that you play with falling in different ways out of balance poses so that balancing becomes a practice of embracing the knowledge that you can fall skillfully and then develop the ability to actually do so.

Additional benefits of a balance practice include developing focus and concentration along with a quieter mind. The self-awareness brought about through a regular balance practice is invaluable, especially as you translate your understanding into daily activities. Balancing poses offer immediate feedback of how the mind–body connection works. If the mind–body complex is disturbed at any level, the instability of that disturbance is immediately reflected back to you in your experience of the pose. When these types of disturbances arise, the practices of identifying, differentiating, and integrating become important components. Apply what you learn about yourself to enhancing your overall life balance. Be compassionate with yourself as you continue to explore new challenges in your balancing—and falling—practice in daily life.

Elements of Balance

1 From standing in mountain pose (next to wall if necessary), lift one foot from an inch to a foot (2.5-30 cm) off the ground, keeping your arms by your sides. Pay attention to the ankle and foot of the standing leg as you begin to explore balancing. What parts of the foot are more or less connected to the ground? How much does the ankle move or not move? Is the foot and ankle rigid and tight or fluid and responsive? Perform the exploration on the other leg. How does the experience vary from side to side?

2 Next exaggerate the movements of the ankle and foot; let them wobble from side to side a bit. Pay attention to the muscles on both sides of the ankle and the lower legs. Can you sense how they adapt with a quick-fire response to this challenge? Notice how this focus changes the experience of balancing. Now try to make the ankle and foot completely rigid and still. What changes? Play around with these concepts as you hold the balance and see whether you can establish an equilibrium between rigidity and fluidity. Do the same thing on the other leg. Again, how does the experience vary from side to side?

3 Start to play with your arm position as you balance on one foot. Try hands on the hips, palms together at heart center, reaching in front of the body, out to the sides at shoulder height, and above the head. What information do the arm positions give you about where your body is in space? Do certain arm positions help you find balance more or less easily than others?

4 Now play with falling out of the one-footed balance. Try falling forward, backward, and sideways. Return to holding the balance. Now play with circling the torso. How far can you lose your balance and still bring yourself back to upright? Regain your balance. How does having strategies for falling affect your experience of holding the pose?

5 Shift your balance exploration to your eyes. Pick one spot at the level of the horizon to softly gaze at. If you are practicing indoors, look for a focal point in the room that is at eye level. Shift your focus to the floor for a bit and then to the ceiling. How does introducing these focal points change your experience of balancing?

6 Hold the balance and try moving the eyes up, down, right, and left without moving the head, neck, or spine. Does the rest of the body want to follow the eyes? Can you differentiate your eye movements from the rest of your body movements and still hold the pose?

7 Now close the eyes completely. Notice how the body wavers as it loses the sense of sight to tell it where it is in space. Stay focused and start to use the arms and legs instead of the eyes to help gather this information. It may seem impossible right now, but with practice you can develop or refine your ability to balance, even with your eyes closed!

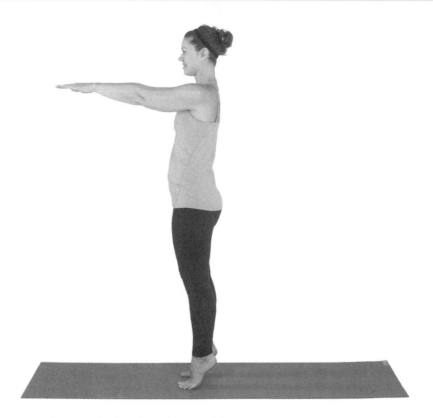

1. Start standing with the feet hip-width apart, arms straight out in front of the body at shoulder height and spine in active neutral.
2. Lift the heels of both feet off the floor and balance on the balls of the feet.
3. Hold for 30 to 60 seconds. To exit the pose, slowly lower the heels back to the floor.

Basic Alternatives

Narrow base: Bring the feet and legs together to touch before lifting the heels off of the ground (a).

Hips externally rotated: Start on a narrow base with the feet on the ground. Move the hips to rotate the heels toward the midline and bring the toes slightly pointing out before lifting the heels off of the ground (b).

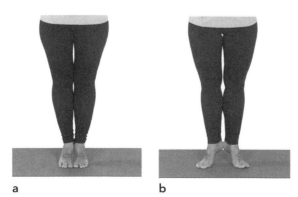

a   b

Block or ball: Hold a small exercise ball or yoga block between the upper thighs, lightly squeezing it throughout the movements and holds *(c)*.

Wall: Start in the basic position with the hands touching the wall before lifting the heels off of the ground *(d)*.

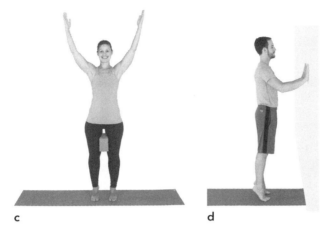

c   d

Mobility Options

Twist: Start in the basic position. Exhale to rotate to the left. Hold for 15 to 60 seconds. Inhale to return to center. Repeat on the other side *(a)*.

Side bend: Start in the basic position with the arms raised overhead. Exhale to arch the torso to the right. Hold for 15 to 60 seconds. Inhale to come back to center. Repeat on the other side *(b)*. This variation can also be done holding a yoga strap drawn taut between the hands.

Backbend: Start in the basic position with the arms raised overhead. Articulate through the midback as you raise the chest skyward. Open the throat slightly, maintaining space and length through the back of the neck. Hold for 15 to 30 seconds *(c)*. This variation can also be done with arms down and behind the body, holding a yoga strap between them and drawn taut.

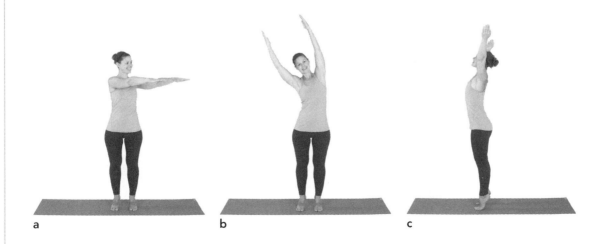

a   b   c

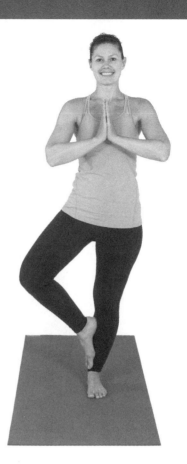

① Start by standing with the palms together in front of the chest.

② Connect all three points of the left foot to the ground. Bend the right knee as you lift the foot off of the ground and open the hip out to the right side. Place the left foot onto the inner left calf. Lightly press the foot into the leg and vice-versa.

③ Hold for 1 to 2 minutes and repeat on the other side.

Basic Options

Foot on the floor: Instead of lifting the right foot off the ground and placing it against the left calf, raise the right heel off of the ground while keeping the ball of the foot on the floor (a).

Foot disconnected from leg: Position the foot of the bent knee 1 to 3 inches (1.3 cm) from the inside of the standing leg instead of touching it (b).

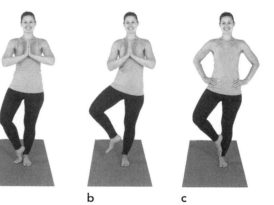

a   b   c

Arms at the hips: Place the hands on the pelvis with the elbows bent and pointing away from the body. Gently press the hands down on the pelvis (c).

Side of the body at the wall: Position yourself so the standing leg is next to the wall. Place the hand of the standing leg side on the wall (d). Arm can be long overhead (as pictured).

Bent knee at the wall: Position yourself so the bent knee leg is next to the wall. Place the block on the low setting (long and flat) between the knee and the wall. Lightly press the knee into the block, maintaining a level pelvis as you hold it there (e).

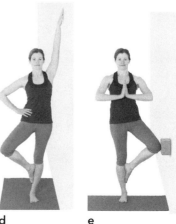

d   e

Mobility Options

Ankle variation 1: Lessen the connection between the foot and leg without completely breaking contact. Let the ankle on the standing leg wobble slightly from left to right.

Ankle variation 2: Stand on one leg on a block on the flat horizontal setting on the floor (a).

Articulating tree: Start in the basic position with the arms out to the sides at shoulder height and hands in gentle fists facing skyward. Exhale and roll the fists downward, initiating the movement from the shoulders and allowing the upper spine to follow into roundness (b). Inhale, rolling the fists away from the floor, initiating the movement from the shoulders as you articulate the spine back through neutral and then into a thoracic-focused backbend (c). Repeat 5 to 10 times.

Twisting tree: Start in the basic position with the hands together in front of the chest. Exhale to rotate through the midtorso to the right. Hold for 15 to 30 seconds. Inhale to return to center and rotate to the left. Repeat standing on the opposite leg (d).

Swaying side-bend tree: Let the upper body sway and arch slowly from side to side to create a flowing side-bend experience (e).

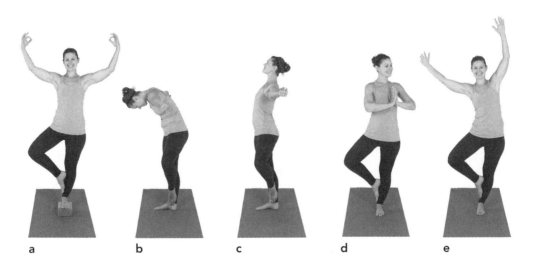

a   b   c   d   e

Recovery Option

Reclined tree: Re-create the tree shape, with the legs in a reclined position, reaching the arms above the head.

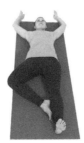

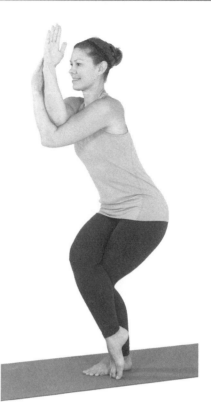

1. Stand with the legs together. Bend both elbows and bring them in front of the body. Shoulder blades spread apart as you crook the right elbow inside the left at the center of the body. Hands can stay apart, or allow the backs of the hands or palms to touch.

2. Bend the knees and sink the hips back into a shallow chair position. Cross the back of the right thigh over the front of the left thigh. Keep the ball of the right foot on the ground as you squeeze the legs together and settle the hips back and down into an asymmetrical squat.

3. Spine stays in active neutral as you hinge slightly forward from the hips to counterbalance the body. Once settled, you can try lifting the right foot from the floor into a single-leg balance.

4. Hold for 30 to 60 seconds and repeat on the other side.

Basic Options

Partial entry: Don't lower down or back as far into the squat (a).

Crossed arms: Cross the arms in front of the body, stacking one on top of the other, then bend the elbows to wrap the hands around the shoulders (b).

Strap: Cross the forearms in front of the body with the palms facing the torso. Hold a strap in both hands and draw it taut (c).

Arms at center: Bring the palms and forearms together in front of the body (d). This variation can be done with the legs crossed, as in the basic pose, or with the figure 4 legs (as pictured).

Foot on block: In the basic position, place the right foot on a block on the floor on its horizontal setting (e).

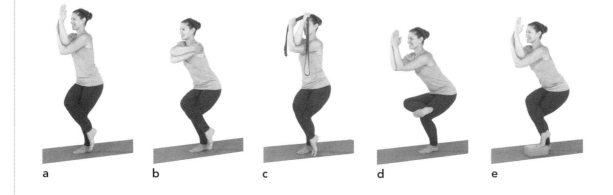

a   b   c   d   e

Figure 4 Legs: Cross the right ankle above left knee, allowing the right hip to externally rotate as you squat *(f)*.

At the wall: Stand with your back about a foot (30 cm) from the wall so that when you squat and the torso moves forward, the buttocks come in contact with the wall *(g)*.

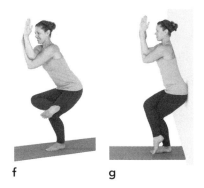

f   g

 ## Mobility Options

Reclined eagle variation 1 (with arm flow): Start in a reclined position with the knees bent and feet on the mat. Bend both elbows and bring them in front of the body. Position the right elbow inside the left at the center of the body. Hands can stay apart, or allow the backs of the hands or palms to touch. Cross the right thigh over the left so that the back of the left thigh is in contact with the front of the right thigh. Keep the right foot on the floor.

Inhale and gently lift the wrapped arms up toward the head. Exhale to bring the arms down toward the chest *(a)*. The spine stays in active neutral as you focus the movement in the shoulders. Repeat 5 to 10 times. Switch arms and repeat on the other side. The arm flow can also be done in the standing variations.

Cat–cow: From the basic standing variation, inhale and lift the arms in front of the face, arching into a slight backbend *(b)*. Exhale and lower the arms toward the chest into a forward bend focused on the upper body *(c)*. Repeat 5 to 10 times, and then repeat on the opposite side.

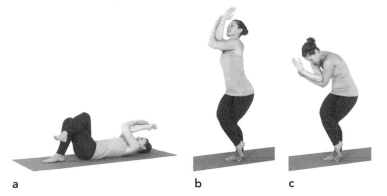

a   b   c

Recovery Option

Reclined eagle variation 2: Start in a reclined position with the knees bent and feet on the mat. Cross the right thigh over the left so that the back of the left thigh is in contact with the front of the right thigh. Bring the legs in toward the torso and hold onto the shins or ankles to secure them into the shape. Use the left hand on the right thigh to gently encourage it towards crossing the midline of the body. Hold for 1 to 2 minutes and repeat on the other side.

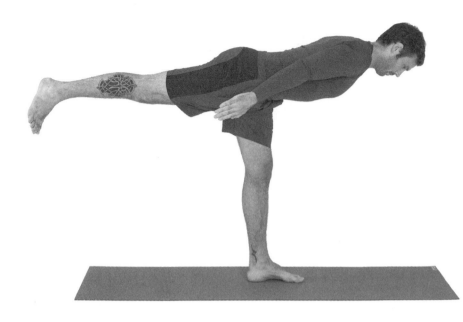

1. Stand with the feet hip-width apart and the arms active along the sides of the body with the palms facing the body. Step the right leg 1 to 3 feet (30-91 cm) behind you, placing the ball of the right foot on the floor.

2. With the spine in active neutral, hinge the torso forward from the front hip, allowing the right foot to lift from the floor as you do so. Bring the torso in line with the floor and the back leg in line with the torso. Flex the back foot. Keep the arms long at the side of the body, actively reaching towards the feet.

3. Hold for 30 to 60 seconds.

Basic Options

Partial entry: Reduce the front-leg hip hinge. Keep the leg in line with the torso, but at a smaller angle in relation to the floor (a).

Bent-knee variation 1: Slightly bend the front leg (b).

Bent-knee variation 2: Bend the back knee anywhere from a small bend to a 90-degree angle (c).

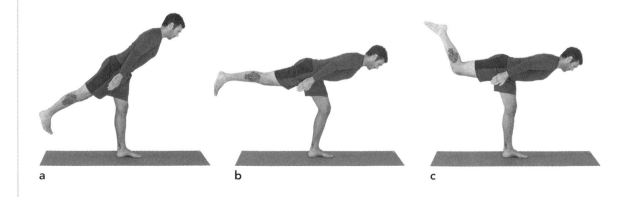

a   b   c

Bent-knee variation 3: Combine variations 1 and 2 bent-leg options *(d)*.

Arms variation 1: Raise the left arm alongside the head and the right arm along the body *(e)*.

Arms variation 2: Position the arms to the sides at shoulder height and palms toward the floor *(f)*.

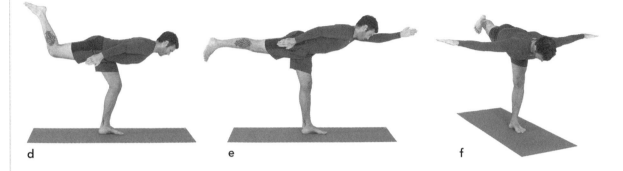

d   e   f

Strength Options

Wall variation 1: Position the arms alongside the ears, and press the hands into the wall *(a)*.

Wall variation 2: Press the back foot into the wall. This is a great variation to explore moving the arms into a variety of positions *(b)*.

Strap pull: Before entering into the pose, position the arms in front of the body with the palms facing forward. Hold a yoga strap or exercise band between the hands and pull it taut as you enter, hold and exit the pose *(c)*.

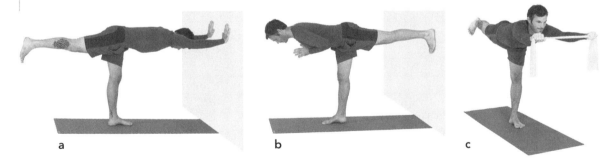

a   b   c

Balance Option

Ball roll: From the basic position, with an exercise ball on the floor in front of the body, place the right hand on the ball and roll it in a small circle. Repeat 5 to 10 times, then circle it in the other direction.

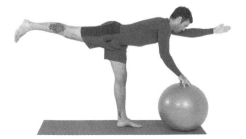

Hips

If you have been in group yoga classes or studied other yoga books, you may have noticed an emphasis on the concept of "hip opening." Traditional asana practices placed a high value on the flexibility of the hips because many yoga poses were employed as a way to prepare the body and mind for meditation. These "traditional" meditative seats required a large a degree of external rotation in the hips. You can see this in some of the older yoga pose texts and even some of the more modern ones. Yet, lotus pose, often called the supreme meditative seat, is not structurally available to a large portion of the population practicing yoga today. For those it is readily available to, it is a fine position to sit in. But the average person exploring the therapeutic benefits of yoga does not need to work toward sitting in lotus because it is neither structurally practical nor is it a requirement for meditation. Meditation is more about a certain state of mind than the ability to sit in a specific shape.

Looking critically at the scope of practices often labeled as hip openers, a pattern emerges: An inordinate number of poses focus on external rotation of the hips. If one of the traditional purposes of asana was to prepare the body and mind to sit in meditation for extended periods, the emphasis on openness starts to makes sense. However, many traditional yogis had different intentions for practice than we do in the modern age, and the traditional emphasis on practices to prepare the body for extended periods of meditation has translated into an impractical tendency in modern styles to favor hip flexibility over hip stability.

An ongoing dialogue about this imbalance in modern yoga practice has caused many yoga teachers and yoga therapists to shift their focus away from the concept of hip opening and toward the concept of hip mobility. While many people in the West do have limited motion in their hips, which could cause them to pursue opening their hips in practice, forcing the hip repeatedly into any extreme position can be counterproductive. A person doesn't really need that much hip flexibility while doing daily activities. Also, the hip stiffness that many people experience has developed over years or decades. In those cases, the capsule around the hip joint has likely lost some pliability and extendibility. This means the space between the bones is narrower, and trying to get into lotus pose or any other position that requires extreme ranges of motion can grind the hip joint into the socket and damage the joint in the long term, especially if the practitioner is using repeated force in her attempt to execute those ranges of motion.

A good rule of thumb to prevent this potential damage in practice is to avoid using the hands or arms to push or pull the hips into a range of motion that cannot be accomplished otherwise. For example, many people reach down to pull their foot up into their groin in tree pose or pull their leg up in the air in standing hand-to-foot pose. While this approach might not be immediately injurious, over time the practitioner can get into a habit of pulling the hips into ranges of motion she does not have the strength to sustain. It is important to explore those poses without the help of the hands for the entry, hold, and exit of the pose.

In previous chapters, we talked about the difference between flexibility and mobility, and we asked that you put any gains that you might make in flexibility through your yoga practice into the context of being able to control the range of motion as it happens. It is worth reminding you of this intention as we approach working with a focus on the hips. A good intention for the hip joint, as for any other joint, is to make sure you are not stronger than flexible or more flexible than strong.

The intention is toward controlled mobility of all your joints, and that includes the hips. You have already been working with the concept of mobility throughout the course of this book and have explored yoga poses that have a hip-mobility component. At this point, you have a sense of how balanced hip joint movement requires a combination of stability, flexibility, and motor control.

Still, it is important for people who experience limited range of motion in their hips to explore the concept of hip mobility in their yoga practice as a way to balance that limited range of motion. If your intention is to relax tight hip muscles, consider using a gentle approach that allows your body to feel safe as you focus on relaxing the nervous system. A less-is-more strategy that is gradual, progressive, responsive, compassionate, and breath-centered will be more effective than one that pushes you to extremes. It will also be helpful for you to explore the variations highlighted in the mobility and recovery sections. The nature of the poses in the recovery section may offer the time and space to process the energetic, emotional, mental, and spiritual patterns that arise as you explore this area of your body, offering fertile ground for a variety of personal inquiries and integrated mind–body understandings.

EXPLORATION

Hip Mobility With Pelvic Stability

❶ Revisit the reclined foot, leg, and hips series from chapter 8, with an emphasis on differentiating your hip movement from your pelvic movement in a variety of orientations. In all of these positions, are you able to keep the pelvis relatively still as you move the hip in the socket?

❷ Now assume a reclined position with the arms by the sides and both legs straight on the floor. Keep the legs relaxed and the feet pointing in a direction that is natural and relaxed for you. Take a couple of breaths and settle into an active neutral spine, keeping equal weight against the floor on both sides of the pelvis.

❸ Inhale and slowly rotate the right leg to the right, so that the foot points out to the right (external rotation). Explore how far you can go before the weight of the pelvis shifts more toward one side or the other (a). Exhale and slowly rotate the leg back through the starting position and in toward the left leg (internal rotation) (b). Are you able to keep the pelvis stable as you move the hip in the socket? Repeat several times on the right leg and then try it on the left leg. How does your experience differ from side to side?

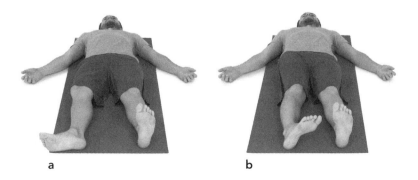

a   b

> continued

4 If you are unable to keep the pelvis stable as the hip moves, try to sense when the pelvic movement happens. Can you make the hip movement smaller and figure out how to stop the hip movement before the pelvis moves? Try this first with the right leg and then with the left. How does your experience differ on each side?

5 Now try starting and finishing the hip movements with the knee bent and foot on the floor, keeping the shin in line with the knee. Again, try it first with the right leg and then with the left. How does your experience differ when the knee is bent instead of straight?

6 Lie with your left side of the body on the floor. Lift the right leg slightly and turn it toward the ceiling (external rotation). Now turn it toward the floor (internal rotation). How does your experience change when your pelvis does not have the support and feedback of the floor? Was it more or less difficult to sense when you had reached the limit of hip movement? Was it more or less difficult to notice when the pelvis started to move? Switch to lying on the right side and rotate the left leg. How does your experience differ on each side?

7 Stand in mountain pose. Put a little more weight on the left leg (c). Reduce the weight on the front of the right foot as you roll through the right hip to move the foot out to the right (external rotation) and then in to the left (internal rotation). Can you keep the right heel still as you pivot on it to move the front of the foot? Can you stop the hip movement before the pelvis moves? Do this several times. Do you have more or less hip movement when standing than you did when you were on your back?

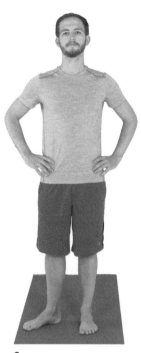

c

8 Now reduce the weight on the heel as you pivot on the front of the foot, sweeping the heel to the right and then to the left. How does the experience of pivoting on the front of the foot differ from pivoting on the heel?

9 Perform the same movements from step 8, but this time allow the pelvis to move with the hip (d). Then hold the pelvis still and allow only the hip to move. Can you feel a difference?

10 Perform the same sequence of movements in steps 7 through 9, but this time put more weight on the right leg and move the left leg and foot. How does your experience differ from side to side?

11 Continue to explore the concept of differentiated hip movement in the poses highlighted in this section. This will be especially interesting in the poses that require more or less muscular activity, as well as poses that ask for spinal positions other than active neutral. See whether you can use what you have learned in this hip exploration to better understand your sensations, achieve subtle nuances in your hip position, and work skillfully to uncover a healthy, sustainable range of motion for your hips.

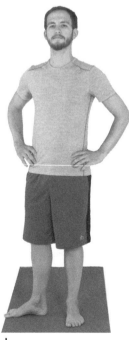

d

Child's Pose

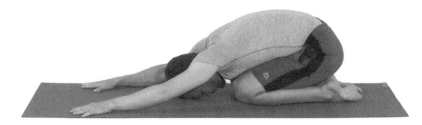

1 Start in table. Lower the buttocks back toward the heels and torso toward the thighs. The arms are straight in front of the body and palms on the mat.

2 Rest the forehead on the floor or a block.

3 Hold for 1 to 3 minutes.

 ## Basic Options

Knees wide option: Widen the knees into a V-shape, shoulders-distance apart or wider, if needed *(a)*.

Blanket option: Tuck a rolled blanket between the back of the upper legs and calves to reduce the amount of knee flexion required *(b)*.

Bolster option: From the knees-wide position, drape the torso over a bolster or large blanket roll. Turn the head to the left or the right so that the side of the face rests on the bolster. If you explore a longer hold, turn the head in the opposite direction mid hold *(c)*.

Ball option: Drape the torso over a large exercise ball and let the arms hang off of it to the sides with the forearms on the ground. Keep the buttocks up and away from the feet. If needed, place the forehead on a block for a more relaxed sense of connection to the floor *(d)*.

Arms by the sides: Roll the upper arms toward the floor and rest the arms on the floor at the sides of the body *(e)*.

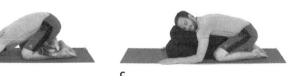

a   b   c

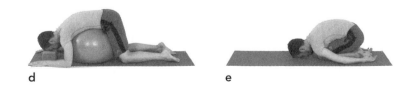

d   e

Mobility Options

Cat–cow: Start with the arms long in front of you and palms on the mat. Spread the knees slightly apart into a V-shape. Exhale to articulate the spine into roundness, allowing the pelvis to lift slightly and the forehead to disconnect from the mat as you go *(a)*. Inhale to reverse the articulation, open the chest, and create a small backbend *(b)*. Repeat 5 to 10 times.

Side bend: Start with the arms out front by the ears, palms or fingertips on the mat and knees together or apart. Walk the arms and torso over to the left side, lengthening through the right side of the body as you arch over to the left. Keep the arms straight, grounding the palms and keeping equal weight into both shins. Hold for 1 to 2 minutes and repeat on the other side *(c)*.

Twist: Start with the arms out front by the ears, palms or fingertips on the mat, knees together or apart. Raise the torso slightly and slide the right arm under the torso at about shoulder level, with the palm facing skyward. Press lightly into the left palm to slightly lift and help rotate the torso to the left. Hold for 1 to 2 minutes and repeat on the other side *(d)*.

Revolved child to table: Start in child's pose with the buttocks back toward the heels. Bring the right hand behind the base of the head and the elbow pointing out to the side *(e)*. Inhale to initiate rotation to the right, shifting the hips up and forward into table pose as you continue to rotate *(f)*. Undo the rotation as you sit the buttocks back toward the heels. Repeat 5 to 10 times on each side.

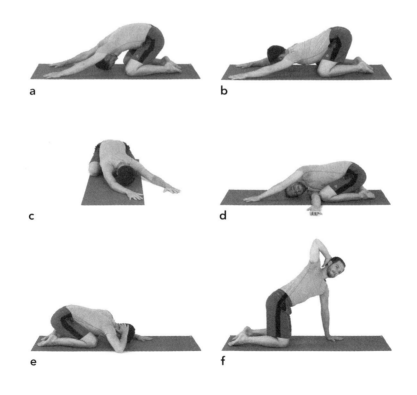

a

b

c

d

e

f

Strength Option

Articulation on the exercise ball: Start in a kneeling table position with the spine in active neutral, arms long by the ears, and hands pressing lightly into a large exercise ball (a). Keep the core active as you exhale to bring the chin toward the chest as you slowly articulate the spine into roundness, rolling the ball toward you as you go (b). Exhale to slowly articulate the spine back through active neutral and then into a small backbend as the ball rolls away from you (c). Repeat 5 to 10 times.

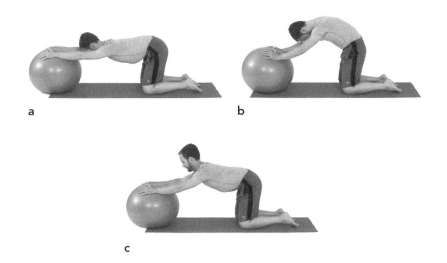

a

b

c

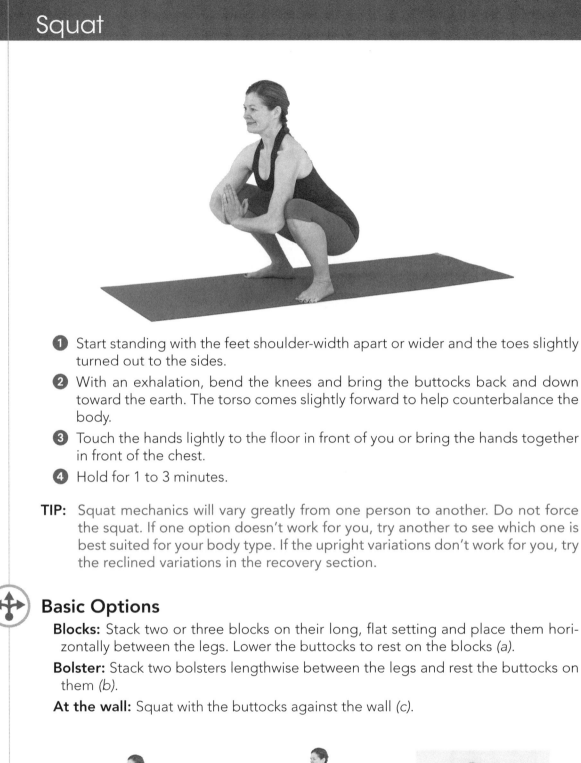

1. Start standing with the feet shoulder-width apart or wider and the toes slightly turned out to the sides.

2. With an exhalation, bend the knees and bring the buttocks back and down toward the earth. The torso comes slightly forward to help counterbalance the body.

3. Touch the hands lightly to the floor in front of you or bring the hands together in front of the chest.

4. Hold for 1 to 3 minutes.

TIP: Squat mechanics will vary greatly from one person to another. Do not force the squat. If one option doesn't work for you, try another to see which one is best suited for your body type. If the upright variations don't work for you, try the reclined variations in the recovery section.

Basic Options

Blocks: Stack two or three blocks on their long, flat setting and place them horizontally between the legs. Lower the buttocks to rest on the blocks (a).

Bolster: Stack two bolsters lengthwise between the legs and rest the buttocks on them (b).

At the wall: Squat with the buttocks against the wall (c).

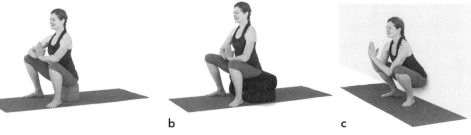

a   b   c

On the chair: Lower the buttocks onto a chair *(d)*.

Blanket variation 1: If the heels don't meet the floor easily, tuck a rolled blanket or pillow under them *(e)*.

Blanket variation 2: To reduce the amount of knee flexion required, tuck a small rolled blanket behind the knees *(f)*.

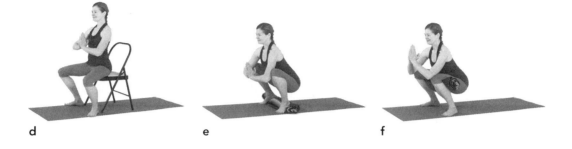

d   e   f

Mobility Options

Forward fold: From the basic or modified position, emphasize rounding the spine forward toward the floor. Walk the hands out and down onto the floor *(a)*.

Twist: From the basic or modified position, bring the right arm inside of the right thigh, with the palm on the floor or a block. Rotate to the left, opening the left arm out straight to the side at shoulder height. Repeat on the other side *(b)*.

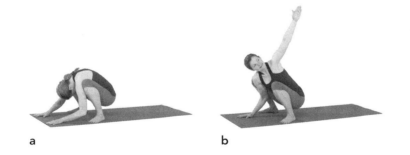

a   b

Recovery Option

Reclined squat at the wall: Start reclined with the knees in toward the chest and the buttocks facing the wall. Bring the feet to the wall and turn them slightly out to the sides. You may need to experiment with how close or far you are from the wall to find a sweet spot for the hold. Choose a position where you can maintain lumbar lordosis. Hold for 1 to 3 minutes.

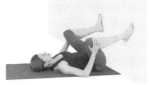

Lunge

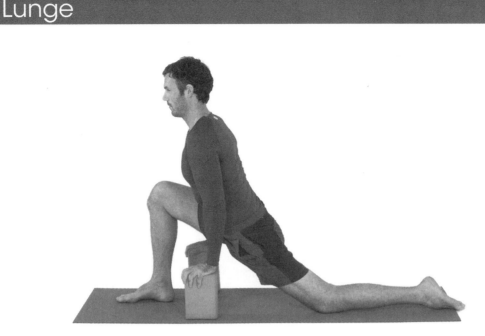

1. Start in a table position with the hands on two blocks on the medium (long and narrow) or high (tall and perpendicular, as pictured) setting.
2. Step the right foot forward. Bend the right knee and align it over the shin and ankle. The left knee and shin are on the ground behind you as you bring the spine into an upright position.
3. Lightly pull the front and back legs toward each other without moving them (as if you were going to pull the mat together) to help create lift in the torso.
4. Hands can stay on the blocks or thigh, or arms can reach up by the ears.
5. Hold for 1 to 2 minutes. Release and repeat with the left leg forward.

Basic Option

Chair: Sit sideways on a chair with the right side of the body toward the chair back and pelvis toward the back of the seat. The right thigh drapes over the chair seat and the right knee is bent and the foot is on the ground or a block. The left leg is off of the chair, reaching back, with the knee bent or the leg long (as pictured) and the ball of the foot on the ground. The right hand is on the chair back and the left arm can stay at the side of the body or reach overhead. Hold for 1 to 2 minutes and repeat on the other side.

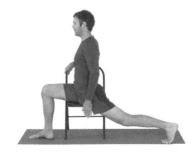

Mobility Options

Forward fold: Start in the basic position and walk the front leg toward the outer edge of the mat 1 to 2 inches in order to accommodate the coming change in spinal position. Round the upper spine toward the floor. Arms can stay straight, or you can walk them inside of the front leg and bend the elbows to place the forearms on the floor, onto blocks *(a)*, or onto a bolster. Hold for 1 to 2 minutes and repeat on the other side.

Backbend: From the basic position, reach the right arm up by the ear as you walk the left hand back to lightly touch the left thigh. Focus on lifting the chest and articulating through the midspine *(b)*. Hold for 1 to 2 minutes and repeat on the other side.

Twist: Start in the basic position and walk the hands up onto the front thigh to help stack the torso over the pelvis. Maintain a stable pelvis as you gently rotate to the left. Bring the right hand to the left thigh and keep the left arm active at shoulder height behind you *(c)*. Hold for 1 to 2 minutes and repeat on the other side.

Side bend: Start in the basic variation with the right leg forward and the spine upright. Lift the left arm by the left ear and arch the spine over to the right into an elongated side bend. Repeat on the other side, with the left leg forward, arching to the left *(d)*.

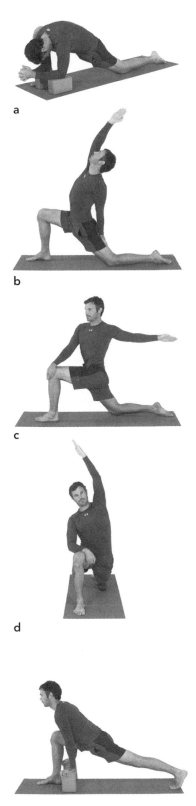

a

b

c

d

Strength Option

Back leg long: Lift the back knee off of the floor to bring the leg straight behind you with the ball of the foot on the ground. Contract the thigh muscles and lightly draw the legs towards each other (as if you were going to pull the mat together) to help support the lift. This variation can be done with hands on the blocks (as pictured), or you can explore more challenges by bringing the arms long and active with the side of the body, or reaching long by the ears.

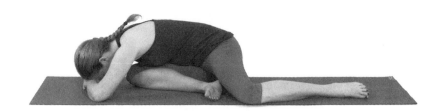

1. Start in a simple, seated position with the legs straight in front of you. Bend the right knee and keep the right leg forward. Sweep the left leg behind the body with the knee bent out to the side.

2. Keep the right hip on the ground as you play with the angle of the thighbone in relation to the pelvis and the distance between the front foot and the groin.

3. Press the hands and fingertips down, while hinging from the hips to angle the spine halfway toward the floor. Stay there, and then with an exhalation, fold over the right leg and rest the forehead on the ground, hands, pillow, block, or bolster.

4. Hold for 1 to 2 minutes and repeat with the left leg forward.

Basic Options

Reclined: Start in a reclined position with both knees bent and both feet on the floor. Cross the right ankle just above the left knee, allowing the hip to externally rotate and the knee to come out to the side.

Reach between the thighs with the right hand and around the outside of the left leg with the left hand to hold the left thigh as you draw it toward the torso only as far as you can while maintaining lumbar lordosis. Hold for 1 to 2 minutes and repeat on the other side (a).

Reclined with a strap: Slide the strap behind the left thigh and hold it in both hands to extend the reach of the arms and allow the upper body to stay on the floor. Repeat on the other side (b).

Reclined using the wall: With the knee bent or leg straight, press the left foot into the wall (c and d).

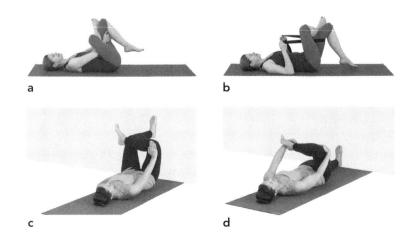

a

b

c

d

Reclined with the foot down: Keep the left foot on the floor or place it on a yoga block (long, flat setting). Use the right hand to gently encourage the right thighbone away from the torso. Repeat on the other side (e).

Reclined leg cradle: Bend both arms. With the palms facing you, cradle the right shin. Keep the bottom foot on the ground as you play with drawing the right leg in. You may also place the bottom leg straight on the ground in this variation (f).

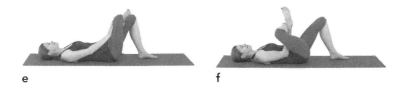

e

f

Mobility Options

Wiggling pigeon: From the basic position, with the spine upright, bring the right foot in toward the groin (a) and lift the right hip off of the floor.

Bring the left leg long behind the body as you activate the hips by attempting to pull the legs toward each other without actually moving them. Press the hands into the floor (b).

Slowly lower the right hip to the right side, stopping short of the floor, and then bring it back to center.

Repeat 5 to 10 times, and then repeat on the other side.

Seated variation 1: Start in an upright seated position with the knees bent and feet on the floor. Create some distance between the torso and thighs. The arms are slightly behind the body with the palms on the ground and elbows bent if needed. Cross the right ankle just above the left knee, allowing the hip to externally rotate and the knee to come out to the side. Repeat on the other side (c).

Seated variation 2: Start in a chair, sitting toward the front edge. Cross the right ankle above the left knee. Try using the right hand to lightly encourage the right thighbone away from the body. Hinge from the hips and fold forward toward the legs. Repeat on the other side (d).

After exploring so many pose variations you might be tempted to think that your journey

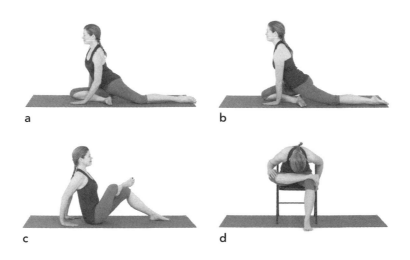

a

b

c

d

of identification, differentiation, and integration ends here. Not so! The options we have outlined here, and the connections that you have made have given you a structural and experiential foundation from which we hope you will continue to build meaningful and effective practice strategies. Your practice will always evolve in response to the phases of your life and how those phases intersect with your changing goals and needs. We have guided your journey up to a certain point, but now it is time for you to take the paths that we have explored together and create a map that is uniquely your own. The next chapter takes a look at where we have been and offers new suggestions for where you might go as you continue to use what you have learned with us to forge a path of inquiry and discovery into other uncharted territories of your mind, body, and spirit. Enjoy your continued journey!

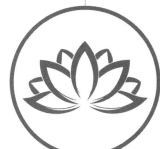

eleven
Maintaining Fitness and Activity Levels

By now it is our hope that you have established a yoga practice and that you have played with some of the concepts we have introduced in this book. The good news is that by using these concepts, you can always find something that will refresh and renew your practice while you continue to learn and adapt. The "bad" news is that there is no end to the ways you can renew your practice. So the responsibility to keep your practice fresh falls on you.

Sometimes it is nice to know that there is an end to what you need to learn and that your practice is set. "This is it. I am done." Feels nice, doesn't it? Just like a diet feels nice because there is an end to it. But lifestyle changes are for life. Our way of practicing is focused on lifestyle change and based on you asking yourself questions such as "What happens if I do this?" Our way of practicing yoga encourages you to continue to play with and change the way you live and look at life.

As you go through life, you will change and so will your practice. There will be days, maybe even weeks, when you will want to do things just the way you have always done them—the familiar way. When your nervous system is overwhelmed by instabilities and life changes, you need the stability and solidity of a familiar asana practice. Follow that voice when you need a break or are overwhelmed. But if that is the message you hear every day, then you need to take a close look at your life to see whether you are really overwhelmed or whether you are just getting into a comfortable, habitual routine. If you are truly overwhelmed, then **identify** what aspects of your life are overwhelming and causing you stress. Then **differentiate** your behaviors in the areas that are overwhelming to you and **integrate** those new behaviors. By all means, take care of yourself and listen to what you need, but when things calm down around you, start playing with your asana practice again. Trust us when we say that we also have times when it is difficult to maintain the freshness and excitement of our practice and when we get stuck in old habits. But we can always ask ourselves, "How can we maintain the freshness, excitement, and joy so that our practice will be lifelong and not end up on the heap of things we have tried and quit?"

Setting Goals for Your Practice

Before we go into how to keep your practice fresh, we will look at what your goals are for your practice. You might think that yoga should not have goals, that yoga exists on a higher plane, or you might have other ideas about what yoga is. This book is about how to use yoga to stay active as you go through life. See, there is a goal right there: to stay active as you go through life. But most of us need goals that are more specific than that. Many times we start yoga, or any personal practice, because there is something that we would like to do well, or there is some aspect of our life that is not working out as well as we would like. Sometimes we might not be aware of what our reasons are right away, but we have a sense that we need to do something different to find fulfillment in how we live. So whether we can or cannot immediately identify them, we all have goals for our practice.

Note that there is a difference between goals and intentions. In chapter 8, we talked about setting an intention, but here we talk about setting goals. What are the differences between the two? Goals tend to focus on the future, something specific that you want to accomplish, and usually have an external, observable, measurable component. You either reach your goal or you don't. An intention is an internal process in the present. The intention is independent of you reaching your goal or not. Your intention for a yoga session might be to feel more peaceful, while the goal for your practice might be to control your anger while at work.

It is important when we set goals that they be reasonable. I (Staffan) would like to run as fast as I did when I was 25, but at this point, I cannot. I have allowed my life to become more complex with work and other responsibilities that I prioritize over running twice daily. We all prioritize, so before you set your goals, be realistic and ask yourself how much time you have to practice. Take a realistic look at your life. Identify the essential activities and prioritize them. What is essential will change during your lifetime, but make sure that what you put in the essential column really is essential to you. Then look at other activities that you perform during the day and differentiate activities that are nonessential and do not add to your life but still take up time and drain your energy. Drop those activities or decrease the amount of time you spend on them. Look at the activities you could perform instead that would enhance your life and move you closer to your goals. Then integrate those activities into your day. Once or twice a year, sit down and go through this cycle of looking at how you spend your time and then adjust accordingly. The development and accomplishment of reasonable goals will also build confidence in your abilities.

You may have fantastic ideas about what you want to accomplish. Great! Keep them, but develop goals that will slowly build your self-confidence. Through continued reflections on what is essential for getting to where you want to be, you can refine and expand your goals to accomplish all the fantastic things you dream of. If you know that you only have so much time for yoga, don't develop a practice that takes twice that amount of time. When you are establishing a practice habit, it is better to develop a short practice and be successful in meeting your goal than to try for a long practice and fail. By successfully establishing a practice, you will be more confident in your abilities. Little by little you will develop a longer, stronger practice that will move you closer to your dreams. As you become more confident, you will also notice that you feel better about yourself and have more energy. That will make it easier to continue practicing.

Still, we all hit a point where our practice runs the risk of becoming habitual and automatic. So let's come back to the question from the beginning of this chapter:

How can we maintain that freshness, excitement, and joy that will foster lifelong practice? One way to keep your practice fresh is to focus on a specific aspect of your practice, even though you are doing the same activity or asana sequence. Based on our own practice and from what we hear from students, here are aspects of a practice that you might want to focus on as a way to keep your practice alive, enjoyable, and relevant to your life.

Some of these concepts have been introduced in chapter 2, but here we look at them through a different lens. We look at the concepts as something you can focus on, both on and off the mat, as a way to enhance your active lifestyle.

Transitions

While holding a yoga pose is relatively stable, but moving from pose to pose is not. In the transition from one pose to another, you find instability and the need to control lots of joints through coordinated muscle activity. From an anatomical and nervous system standpoint, you are at a higher risk of injury when you move from pose to pose than when you remain in a static pose. Often when you practice your asana sequence, your focus jumps to the posture you are moving toward. Once in the new asana, you might spend time finding the right alignment, taking a few breaths, and then your mind again is on to the next asana. Many teachers will tell you how to align yourself in the pose. They might even help you find the pose, but seldom do they tell you how to or help you transition from pose to pose. They miss the important part of how you got there: the transition phase from one asana to the next. Instead of focusing on the asanas, try to focus on the transitions between them. How do you get from one asana to the next?

Go back to the concepts of identification, differentiation, and integration. By focusing on one of those phases as you move from one asana to the next, you are coming back to the present moment. Don't let your mind jump to the next asana; instead focus on the transition. Identify how you transition. What part of your body moves first? Do you move on the inhalation or exhalation? Is the transition smooth or do you lose your balance or control at some point during the transition? Then differentiate: Perform the transition in a different way and allow the nervous system to integrate the differentiations into your practice.

Can you sense that when you focus on how you do your transitions, your mind tends to stay in the present and not jump to the asana you are transitioning into? Of course, you can play with any transition, including transitions that are off the yoga mat. How do you transition out of bed in the morning? How do you transition into and out of your car? How do you transition in your thoughts when you go from home to work and from work to home? Your whole life can be described as a series of transitions: infancy to youth to adolescence to adulthood. How do you learn to transition with presence, grace, and agility?

Have fun practicing the yoga transitions while noticing how they may spill over into the transitions you go through during life. By identifying and differentiating the transitions and then taking them into daily life, you are integrating what you learn on the mat into your life. That is real integration. Once you notice real integration, your practice will be immensely more interesting because you will clearly see how your practice influences your life. You will be amazed at the changes you notice, and those changes will provide inspiration to your practice.

Transition 1

1 Stand in mountain. Go into warrior 1 and then transition into warrior 2. How did you do that? Do it one more time and pay attention to what moves first when you go from mountain to warrior 1.

2 Three things could move first: the legs and pelvis, the arms, or the head. What moves first when you transition from mountain to warrior 1? From warrior 1 to warrior 2? From warrior 2 to warrior 1, and back to mountain?

3 Once you have identified how you habitually start the movement, try something different. How does the movement change if you initiate with the legs instead of the arms or the head instead of the arms? With what other parts could you initiate the movement? Could you even initiate the movement with your eyes?

4 Start in mountain as before, but now pay attention to your breath. Do you start the transition on the inhalation or exhalation? Now reverse, or differentiate, it. If you start on the inhalation, start the movement on the exhalation. This forces you to use your muscles and nervous system differently because on the inhalation, the body expands and the muscles are ready for action. On the exhalation, the body relaxes and the muscles are not quite as ready for action.

Agility in Transitions

Watch students go through a sequence of yoga poses. While they all might look great once they are in the poses, some students appear to float from pose to pose. Others have trouble moving smoothly and may struggle as they transition between poses. Agility might be one of the most overlooked benefits of yoga asana practice. The reason is that the focus tends to be on the pose and not the transition from pose to pose.

The following explorations require agility. You can always make the transitions more elegant, more efficient, and more agile. More agility in transitions between poses means that you are better able to control your movements. This will lead to more enjoyment and decrease the risk of injuries during yoga practice and during other activities you enjoy.

In the following explorations, pay as much, if not more, attention to the transition from pose to pose as you do to the pose itself. Instead of paying attention to the concepts that we introduced in the previous section on transitions, pay attention to applying aspects of agility and grace. We spoke about some of these aspects of agility in chapter 2. We will reintroduce some of the same concepts here, but now in the context of agility during transitions.

Falling in Transitions

Don't "fall" into your next pose as you transition from one into another. For example, it is common to fall onto the back leg when stepping back from mountain to warrior 1. To develop agility, work on maintaining your balance at all times, even during transitions. In the case of moving from mountain to warrior 1, determine how far you can step back with the leg without falling onto the back foot. This position allows you to step back into mountain when you are finished with your warrior series without having to lunge forward or use a lot of force to return to mountain. There are times in yoga when you transition by jumping or making other fast movements, but to train agility and control, you should perform the transitions slowly from pose to pose, always maintaining balance and control of your movements.

Making Transitions Reversible

To make your movements reversible, be sure you can stop the transition into a pose and return to the pose you were transitioning out of. Initially, you will most likely have to shorten your step back into warrior, narrow your stance in triangle, and adjust your lunges. However, as your agility and movement control increase, your poses will look and feel like they used to. The difference is that the improved agility and control of your movements will decrease your risk of injury. Your sequences will "float" and be more enjoyable because you are in control of your movements.

Staying Grounded in Transitions

Use the ground. We have talked about the importance of being aware of the three points of the foot—base of the big toe, base of the pinky toe, center of the heel—for balance and grounding. When working on agility, you will learn how to use the ground and how to push off from those three points. Many transitions require a change in how you bear weight on your hands and feet. You might have to put more weight on one foot than the other, lift one foot from the ground while staying grounded on the other, or push off with one foot or hand while putting more weight on the other foot or hand.

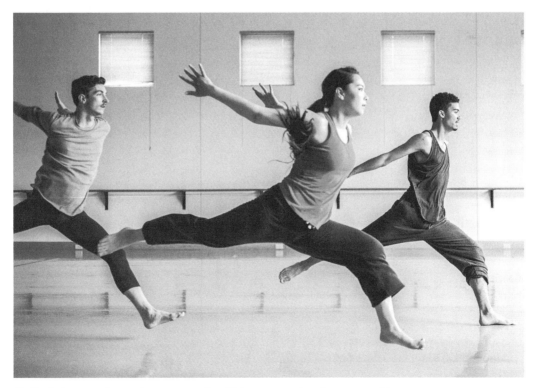

Skilled dancers know how to push off the ground to become airborne.

EXPLORATION
Transition 2

1 Stand in mountain. Go into warrior 1 and then transition into warrior 2. How did you do that? Do it one more time and pay attention to whether you "fall" when you step back from mountain to warrior 1. If you fall as you step back, your transition is not reversible. Try to shorten the step back from mountain to warrior 1.

2 From warrior 1, step forward to mountain. Was the transition back to mountain smooth and reversible throughout, or was there a moment in the transition where you lost control of the movement and had to use momentum and force to come back to mountain?

3 Return to mountain. Transition from mountain to warrior 1, then to warrior 2, and then back to mountain. Were you aware of how you used the ground? Do the same sequence again, but push from the ground when you transition. Pay attention to the three points that ground the foot: big toe, little toe, center of heel. Are you pushing off from all three?

4 Try to push off from different parts of the foot as you transition and then go back to pushing from the three points. Go through the sequence again, but this time try not to push from the floor. Instead, lift more as you transition. Did that make the sequence easier or did you have to use more muscular effort? Then do the initial sequence and see how the movement has changed as the nervous system has integrated all the movement options that you explored.

Watch accomplished dancers and notice how they appear to float through the air. Notice that before they are able to float, they push off from the ground. If you want to move forward, you have to push back. If you want to move up, you have to push down. Too often we forget these basic ideas from physics. To improve your agility, you need to think about how to use the ground when you move. Identify how you use the ground when you move from one pose to the next. How do you use your hands and feet to push off from the ground? Do you push off? Differentiate and use the ground in a different way. Did that change your transition? Did the movement become more reversible? Did it feel safer? More elegant?

When you perform the following sequences, play with these concepts. Are you in control of your movements? Are your movements reversible? How are you using the ground?

How much effort do you use when you are playing tennis, getting out of bed, walking, or rising from sitting to standing? If you use the ground differently, does that make your activities different, more or less effortless or elegant? An activity performed with agility is usually more effortless and elegant. Do you feel elegant when you are on the mat or when you perform activities during your normal day? Are your activities reversible? When you move from sitting to standing, or from standing to sitting, do you use momentum or let gravity pull you down into the chair? How can you perform those activities with reversibility so that you do not fall those last few inches when you are about to sit on the chair?

Transferring Agility to Daily Life

Most people want to stay active throughout their lives. An important factor in staying active is to avoid injuries. Injuries slow you down and force you to rest or to modify your activities. As you age, your ability to remain active becomes more and more important. Most of the changes blamed on aging are more likely the result of the more sedentary lifestyles that many people adopt as they age. We claim that we deserve to take it easier as we get older. If anything, we should probably try to stay even more active as we age. So how does working on transitions and agility help us off the mat?

When you focus on agility in your asana practice, simultaneously focus on agility in your daily life. Every activity that you perform, whether it is playing tennis, getting out of bed, walking, or getting out of a chair, involves periods of stability and instability. In daily life, just as in yoga, people tend to focus on the action they are about to do. In tennis, they focus on hitting the ball. When getting out of bed, they focus on what they will do once they are standing. In rising from sitting to standing, they focus on the standing. When you miss the transitions, you tend to get injured or fall in the transition phase. We suggest that just like you focus on transitions in your asana practice, try to focus and play with transitions in your daily activities as much as on the final activity itself.

Working on transitions and agility in asana practice is also beneficial if you lose your balance or fall. Losing your balance is really just another transition. Having practiced transitions, reversing movements, using the floor, and knowing where your limbs and spine are in space will help you find a way to lose your balance with grace and elegance. Your chance of getting injured will decrease if you lose your balance with grace and elegance. If you use these concepts and practices of transitions and agility on and off the mat, you will more than likely notice that you perform your activities with more efficiency and enjoyment. Proprioception is one more aspect of asana practice that you can play with to get ready for a more active and enjoyable lifestyle.

Asana Practice for the Proprioceptors

Proprioception is the sense of where the body is in space and the sense of effort and movement. Proprioception greatly contributes to the sense of balance. A variety of proprioceptors exist throughout the body: inner ear, muscles, tendons, joints—just about everywhere. The brain collects the information from the proprioceptors and then creates a map of where the body is in space. From that map, the brain sends commands to the muscles regarding what action they should perform. One can say that the nervous system tries to create an appropriate response to a situation based on the information it receives from the proprioceptors and other senses. The nervous system incorporates previous information and experiences with the new information to create the response.

Of course, this is a simplified description of what happens in the nervous system when it gets information from the proprioceptors. What is interesting and often overlooked about the way the nervous system creates a response is that the responses are based on past experiences. This means that if you always do yoga with the proprioceptors "lined up," then when you are not aligned, the nervous system will not react as fast, or know how to produce the right response, sometimes causing you to fall or injure yourself. So how do you train your nervous system to be ready to respond when the proprioceptors are misaligned or when the message to the nervous system does not look like anything it has experienced before?

EXPLORATION

Proprioception

1 Stand in mountain. Go into warrior 1, and then transition into warrior 2. What was your head position as you moved from asana to asana? In both warrior 1 and 2, the head is usually positioned so you can gaze forward. The eyes look in the direction of the front hand and foot.

2 Now perform the same sequence, but look to the right as you step back with the right foot into warrior 1 (a). Then look to the left as you do the sequence on the left (b). Now reverse it. Look to the left as you do the sequences, stepping back on the right foot as you transition into warrior 1. Then look right as you do the sequence on the left.

3 To make it more interesting for your proprioceptors, can you rotate your head from side to side throughout the sequence? Can you tilt your head from side to side? Look up at the ceiling?

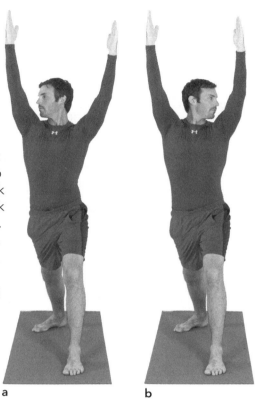

a   b

Asana practice trains your nervous system to recognize when your proprioceptors are not aligned and then to respond appropriately. When you go into downward dog, triangle, eagle, or other asanas, you are training your nervous system to respond to information from the proprioceptors that it may not immediately recognize. Again, we are coming back to the idea of creating puzzles for the nervous system. Once you have gone through asana practice for a while, though, it does not offer the same challenge to the nervous system. The nervous system knows that puzzle. You don't do the same jigsaw puzzle over and over again, do you? It gets boring after a while. With some imagination and creativity, you can use the same asanas and sequences and still teach the nervous system to recognize and respond to new patterns of proprioception.

How does proprioception transfer off the mat? Let's use tennis as an example. Unless you are very fast, there will be times when you are out of the optimal position to hit the ball. If you always hit the ball in practice from the perfect position, your nervous system will not be able to react fast enough when you are out of the ideal position, and you will not be able to hit a winner. To play with proprioception in tennis, you might decide to hit the ball with more weight on the front foot, back foot, foot closest to the ball, foot farthest from the ball, and so on. Of course, this will be done in small doses during controlled practice situations and not during matches, but the skills learned during these controlled practices will transfer to your match play.

If you want to practice proprioception for getting in and out of a chair, you might get up with the right leg in front of the left and then the left in front of the right. Most of us prefer to keep one leg in front of the other when we stand up. Again it comes down to identifying your favored leg, then differentiating and putting the other leg in front when you stand, and finally integrating what the nervous system has learned. Instead of playing with different foot positions, you can play with the position of the head. Stand up while looking forward, then hold the head to the left and to the right and then finally stand up while turning your head to the right and left. We're sure that you can come up with many more activities to challenge the nervous system and thereby improve your ability to stay active off the mat by focusing on and playing with the transitions in asana, agility, and proprioception.

Staying Active Throughout Life

We hope you bought this book because you want to stay active for as long as possible and get as much enjoyment as possible from your activities. Throughout you have read about the importance of varied movements and movement explorations. You have read about the benefits of all this, but perhaps you are still unsure of how our approach to yoga and movement is beneficial to your ability to remain active throughout life. So let's review and clarify some of the benefits that you can gain from playing with the concepts in this book.

Final Words on Identifying, Differentiating, and Integrating

Our intention in writing this book has been to introduce you to yoga therapy and how you can use it to continue to live actively throughout your life. We have introduced you to a variety of yoga asanas and variations on the asanas. We believe that while it is not easy to maintain an active lifestyle in today's society, it can be done. More information than ever before is available through the Internet and various publications. Most cities offer yoga classes in a variety of styles. Choose the style and the teacher that meets your needs. No matter what style you choose and what activities you prefer, the concepts of identification, differentiation, and integration will make your yoga practice and chosen activity more enjoyable and satisfying. We have taken you through various asanas and sequences using those concepts, but that is just the beginning of how you can use those concepts in yoga therapy to enhance your life.

Yoga therapy also includes your thoughts, relationships, work, nutrition, and spiritual life. You can play with all those aspects using the concepts in this book. Identify your food habits, relationship habits, work habits, thoughts, and excuses. Once you have identified your habits and habitual responses, differentiate. Eat something different. Respond differently to challenges at work. Respond in a different way to your partner and friends. Respond differently when you have cravings for junk food. Respond differently to habitual ways of living that you want to change. Once you have differentiated, integrate the new responses. Integration means you have options for how to respond. You can respond in a habitual or nonhabitual way. The more ways you can respond to situations in your life, the more successful you will be in adapting to a changing world. So while the ideas that we have presented in the previous chapters will enable you to have a more active and enjoyable life-style, it will also allow you to transform all aspects of your life if you just decide to **identify, differentiate,** and **integrate.**

Good luck!